operative
ultrasonography

operative
ultrasonography

BERNARD SIGEL, M.D.

Professor of Surgery,
University of Illinois College of Medicine,
Chicago, Illinois

Illustrated by:
Russell K. Pearl, M.D.
Instructor in Surgery,
University of Illinois College of Medicine,
Chicago, Illinois

Philadelphia • 1982

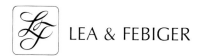
LEA & FEBIGER

Lea & Febiger
600 Washington Square
Philadelphia, PA 19106
U.S.A.

Library of Congress Cataloging in Publication Data

Sigel, Bernard, 1930-
　　Operative ultrasonography.

　　Bibliography: p.
　　Includes index.
　　1. Ultrasonics in surgery. I. Pearl, Russell K.
II. Title. [DNLM: 1. Ultrasonics—Diagnostic use.
2. Surgery, Operative. WO 500 S575o]
RD33.7.S53　　　617'.07543　　　81-18599
ISBN 0-8121-0837-X　　　AACR2

PRINTED IN THE UNITED STATES OF AMERICA

Print No. 3 2 1

To Lois Savitch Sigel

PREFACE

Operative ultrasonography is the application of ultrasound scanning techniques during surgical operations. Since this involves identification and selection of appropriate tissues and the placement of sterile ultrasound instruments in direct contact with organs and tissues, the surgeon is the individual who must perform the procedure. This book is for the surgeon who is interested in using imaging ultrasound in the operating room.

The intent of this book is to accomplish three objectives. The first is to familiarize surgeons with the principles of ultrasound, with the terminology, and with the reasons behind the specific applications. The second objective is to describe the instruments and techniques as used in the operating room. This will consider the details of how ultrasonography is used in conformance with the requirements and limits imposed by the operation. The final objective is to describe the specific applications of operative ultrasonography. Four major applications of operative ultrasound are described in detail. These are the uses of ultrasound during biliary, pancreatic, renal, and vascular surgery. Other uses of operative ultrasound for which there is yet limited experience are briefly summarized. These include localization of foreign bodies, utilization in brain surgery, detection of solid organ abscesses, and detection of endocrine tumors.

One of the first steps necessary in performing operative ultrasonography is to establish a working relationship with the radiologist or ultrasonographer who is expert in this field. This is essential. There must be the same collaboration as exists in the performance of operative cholangiography, pancreatography, urography, and arteriography. The relationship between the surgeon and ultrasonographer may vary from the surgeon interpreting the images and using the ultrasonographer as back-up consultant to the ultrasonographer coming into the operating room for each ultrasonic reading. These relations must be specially tailored to fit individual interests and availability.

vii

It is my hope that this book may provide the surgeon with sufficient information to get started with using ultrasound during surgical procedures. Ultrasound may assist the surgeon in many ways. As with other techniques, ultrasonography requires experience until sufficient dexterity and confidence is developed. Once obtained, the surgeon's tasks in managing certain problems may be greatly facilitated, and this technique may join other diagnostic procedures that have made surgical practice safer and more effective.

My own interest in operative ultrasonography began in 1978. I soon discovered that there had been earlier efforts to apply both A-mode and B-mode ultrasound imaging during surgical procedures. To gain some personal experience and test the potential for using this methodology in biliary surgery, we performed a preliminary series of experiments in animals. This showed the feasibility of using B-mode real-time imaging to locate biliary calculi by direct contact scanning of exposed structures in an operative field.[1] From this, we went to operative application and expanded our field of interest to include a number of different areas in surgery. This experience is the basis for this book.

Whatever achievement I may have made in operative ultrasonography could not have been possible without guidance, teaching, help, and support from many individuals. These include George L. Popky and Dimitrios G. Spigos, both radiologists, who encouraged me to start this venture and who taught me a great deal about ultrasound. I appreciated the support of the High Stoy Technological Corporation, in particular the vision and decisiveness of its Board Chairman, Peter M. Detwiler. Peter Detwiler assumed the risks of a new venture and was the first industrial leader to make a major commitment to operative ultrasound. Jeff Justin, bioengineer, provided important support in both research and clinical application. I gratefully acknowledge the involvement of my surgical colleagues and co-workers: Sabas F. Abuabara, Robert J. Baker, John A. Barrett, C. Thomas Bombeck, Philip E. Donahue, D. Preston Flanigan, Olga M. Jonasson, Avram R. Kraft, Colathur K. Palani, Kevin C. Pringle, Hernan M. Reyes, James J. Schuler, Roohallah Sharifi, William D. Soper, Miguel Teresi, José M. Velasco, W. Bedford Waters, and Donald K. Wood. Julio C.U. Coelho, Surgical Fellow, provided invaluable assistance by working closely with me to develop operative ultrasound. My special thanks go to Christine M. Saliga-Sullivan, my secretary, who not only typed the various drafts of the manuscript but also did a superb job in researching and referencing the illustrative material. I was fortunate to have Russell K. Pearl, Instructor in Surgery, do the illustrations. Finally, and with gratitude, I wish to mention the help and support of Lloyd M. Nyhus, Head of Surgery at Illinois. Lloyd Nyhus instantly recognized the potential of operative ultrasound and did much to make its development possible.

Chicago, Illinois

Bernard Sigel

CONTENTS

Chapter 1 . . . Basics of Ultrasound   1

Chapter 2 . . . Instrumentation 25

Chapter 3 . . . General Techniques 39

Chapter 4 . . . Ultrasonography During Biliary
Tract Surgery 53

Chapter 5 . . . Ultrasonography During Pancreatic
Surgery 85

Chapter 6 . . . Ultrasonography During Renal
Surgery 121

Chapter 7 . . . Ultrasonography During Vascular
Surgery 135

Chapter 8 . . . New and Developing Uses for
Operative Ultrasonography 165

References 181

Index 183

CHAPTER **1**
BASICS
OF
ULTRASOUND

Recent advances in technology make possible the use of ultrasound during surgical procedures. These advances have led to the development of relatively small and simple-to-operate instruments that can display instant motion and high-resolution images of structures encountered during an operation. To most effectively use and interpret ultrasound in the operating room, one must understand some of the basic principles of ultrasonography in general. This chapter is a brief review of selective information that has a direct bearing on the surgical application of ultrasonography. A more comprehensive presentation of the fundamentals of ultrasonography may be found in books dealing with the physics of diagnostic ultrasound.[2,3]

PROPERTIES AND DEFINITIONS

Sound is mechanical energy propagating through a medium as pressure waves. These pressure waves are produced by oscillations of particles within the medium around a sound source and consist of alternating regions of relative compression and rarefaction. Such oscillations propagate in several ways away from the sound source. The most important way, from the standpoint of diagnostic ultrasound, is by means of longitudinal waves.

A longitudinal wave (Fig. 1-1) moves in the same direction as do the back-and-forth oscillations produced by the sound source. Many factors related to the sound source and medium determine the properties of longitudinal waves. The most elementary properties are frequency, propagation velocity, and wavelength.

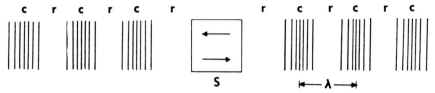

Fig. 1–1. Schematic representation of longitudinal sound waves. A vibrating sound source (S) produces condensations (c) and rarefactions (r) in the surrounding medium. These are pressure waves that propagate away from the source. The distance between two similar points in the wave cycle is the wavelength (λ).

The frequency (f) of the sound is the number of compressions and rarefactions produced in a given time interval. It is usually measured as cycles per second. The frequency unit, defined as one cycle per second, is called the hertz, and its symbol is Hz. This unit is used with the appropriate metric prefix to indicate 1000 (kilohertz, kHz) or 1,000,000 (megahertz, MHz) cycles per second. The frequency of the sound is determined by the frequency of the mechancial vibrations produced by the sound source.

Audible sound is in the frequency range of 20 Hz to 20 kHz. Sound with a frequency above 20 kHz is defined as ultrasound.

The propagation velocity of the sound waves (c) is controlled by the surrounding medium. The medium factors most involved in determining sound propagation velocity are elasticity and density. They relate to velocity as follows:

$$c = \sqrt{\frac{e}{\rho}}$$

Elasticity (e) is the internal force of a medium, which tends to restore deformity produced by an outside force back to its original configuration. It exerts a binding effect on the medium. Density (ρ) is mass per unit volume of a substance. The velocity of sound propagation varies through various media:

air	330 meters/sec
water	1480 meters/sec
soft tissue	1540 meters/sec
bone	3500 meters/sec

Often, the elasticity is the more important factor in determining velocity. For example, in comparing the velocity of sound propagation in air with that in water, velocity is less in air than in water even though the density of air is less. However, the elasticity of water is proportionately much greater, thereby producing the higher velocity.

The wavelength (λ) is the distance between similar locations in the sound wave cycle. These may be measured between points of compression or rarefaction (see Fig. 1-1). The wavelength is determined by the frequency (f) and propagation velocity.

$$\lambda = \frac{c}{f}$$

This equation describes the relationship between the elementary properties of sound. These elementary properties determine a number of other properties related to the transmission and interaction of sound within a medium.

TRANSMISSION AND INTERACTION OF A SOUND IN A MEDIUM

Sound has a number of properties characteristic of energy that propagate in wave form. Some of these properties that relate to the transmission and interaction of sound in a medium are described in terms most applicable to the use of ultrasound in medical diagnosis.

Directionality

Directionality is the ability to beam sound waves along a selected course. This ability varies with the shape and size of the sound source and with the frequency of the produced sound. Longitudinal sound waves tend to spread more at low frequencies than at higher frequencies. Absorptive material attached to the back of the transducers prevents undesired multidirectional spread of sound waves and enhances directionality (Fig. 1-2). Absorptive backing also inhibits reflection of sound beams from the back surface of the

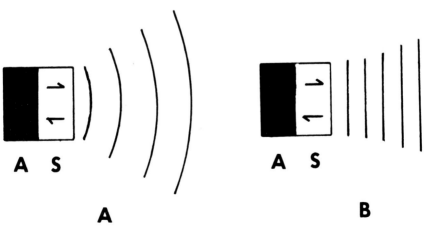

Fig. 1–2. Schematic representation of the effect of frequency on the spread of longitudinal waves. In A, the frequency is low with a corresponding divergency of the sound beam. In B, the frequency is high with a narrower sound beam. Waves are emanating from only one side of the sound source (S). Absorbent backing (A) is placed behind the sound source to prevent reflection of sound from the back wall of the sound source.

sound source that may otherwise propagate outward and complicate the sound beam. The higher the frequency, the easier it is to beam sound waves. In the ultrasound range, particularly at megahertz levels, sound beams remain quite narrow over relatively long distances (see *Transducer Function,* this chapter).

Specular Reflection and Scattering

Beamed ultrasonic waves behave in a manner similar to light. As with light, ultrasound interacting with an object in its path may undergo reflection.

Reflection is the feature on which most of diagnostic ultrasound is based. The sound waves may be directed back toward the sound source in two ways: specular reflection and scattering. The factor that determines which

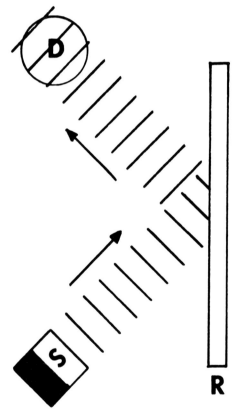

Fig. 1–3. Schematic diagram of specular reflection. A narrow sound beam produced by a sound source (S) is reflected by a smooth barrier (R), which is of considerably larger dimension than the wavelength of the sound. The reflected sound continues as a narrow beam. A sound detector (D) must be in the path of the reflected sound waves to sense the sound signal.

will occur is the relation of the wavelength of the sound to the size of the reflector in the sound beam.

Specular reflection occurs when the sound waves propagating through one medium strike an object or surface of a different medium with a dimension that is larger than the wavelength of the sound beam. The specular reflection of sound from a relatively large, smooth plane surface is similar to the reflection of light by a polished mirror. The angle of reflection is equal to the angle of incidence, and the detector of a reflected beam must be positioned in the line of reflection to sense the beam (Fig. 1-3).

Scattering occurs if the object or surface of a different medium is of a smaller dimension than the wavelength of the incident sound beam. With scattering, sound waves are sent in all directions, and some return in the direction of the sound source (backscattering). Scattering may be produced by small objects in the sound beam, such as blood cells suspended in plasma. Scattering may also occur from the surface of an irregular plane (Fig. 1-4). In this instance, the surface irregularities must be relatively small and multiple. If there are significant large areas of smooth surface, specular reflection will occur. Because of the multiple directions taken, scattered sound energy may be directed over a wide range. Such multidirectional spread weakens the sound intensity in any given direction compared to specular reflection along the single path of the reflection angle.

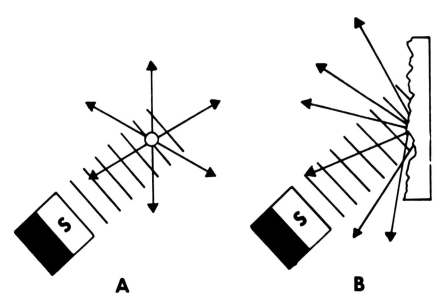

A   **B**

Fig. 1–4.   Schematic diagrams of scattering. In *A*, scattering is produced by a small object. In *B*, scattering is produced by an irregular surface. In both instances, a narrow sound beam (S) is scattered in all directions by reflective objects or surfaces with dimensions that are less than the wavelength of the incident sound.

Refraction

Refraction occurs when propagation waves pass from one medium into another and change direction in the second medium to a course that differs from the original incidence path. Two conditions are necessary for refraction to occur. First, the angle of incidence must be other than 90° in respect to the surface. If the incident beam to the surface is normal, propagating waves will be either reflected and/or transmitted straight through the medium. Second, the velocities of propagation in the two media must be different.

In imaging ultrasound, the source of sound waves is usually also the receptor for reflected waves. For reflection to occur, the source-receptor must be at or near to a right angle to the reflector. Thus, refraction is not a factor in tissue imaging using normal specular ultrasonic reflection. Refraction is an important factor, however, in developing and shaping sound beams that are directed into tissue (see *Transducer Function,* this chapter).

Interference

The interaction of waves on each other is termed interference. This interaction is the sum of the directed energies or particle oscillations of the sound waves. In Figure 1-5, two sound waves of the same frequency are shown in sinusoidal wave form. The sinusoidal wave is a convenient way to depict the strength and direction of particle oscillation in respect to time. This is termed the phase display. A complete wave cycle of 360° or 2π radians represents all the directions of particle oscillation or energy of a

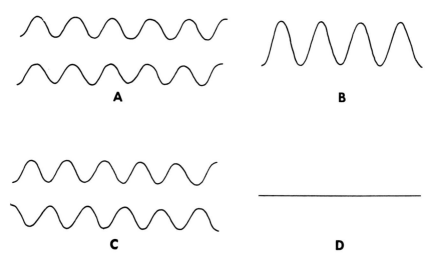

Fig. 1–5. Diagrammatic illustrations of wave interference. Waves are shown in sinusoidal form, which depicts the velocity of particles moving in the pressure oscillation comprising the sound wave. In *A,* two waves are completed in phase. The sum of this interaction is shown in *B,* which depicts a sine wave of greater magnitude. This is reinforcement. In *C,* 2 waves are 180° or completely out of phase. The "peak" of one wave corresponds to a "valley" of the other wave. The sum of corresponding energies that are in opposite directions is zero (*D*). This is cancellation.

longitudinal sound wave. In a complete cycle starting at zero energy, the phase display shows an increase in positive (forward) movement, which peaks and then decreases to zero energy. Particle oscillation passes through the zero level and continues as negative (backward) movement. A negative peak is reached, and the cycle is completed by a return to zero energy. This type of back-and-forth oscillation is called simple harmonic motion.

The phase relation of sound waves determines the type of interference produced by their interaction. Phase relation refers to the points on the wave cycle that correspond to each other at a given time. When positive and negative peaks correspond exactly, the waves are in phase. When two sound waves are in phase, the overall effect is the sum of the energy magnitudes (amplitude and direction) of the waves. This type of interference is termed reinforcement and is a means by which multiple weak waves may produce strong oscillations that can propagate through the media. When the waves are completely out of phase, the energy directions are opposite to each other, and one wave tends to nullify the other. This interference is termed cancellation. Reinforcement and cancellation occur to varying degrees and are related to the amplitude, frequency, and phase relationships of two or more waves that are interacting.

Wave interference is an important feature in the development of ultrasonic signals. Sound sources produce sound waves at multiple points of origin. These multiple waves, through the process of reinforcement, produce the stronger signals that propagate away from the sound source as though they were initiated as a single wave. This is called Huygen's principle and explains the behavior of transducers used in diagnostic ultrasonography.

PIEZOELECTRIC TRANSDUCERS

A transducer is a substance or device that transforms one form of energy into another. Modern diagnostic ultrasound was made possible by development of the piezoelectric transducer, which transforms electrical energy into mechanical energy and the reverse—mechanical energy in the form of sound into electricity.

The piezoelectric effect is a property inherent in certain substances with a crystal lattice structure. When an electric field is applied to the crystal, its shape changes. Conversely, mechanically altering the shape of the crystal generates a weak electric current (Fig. 1-6). Thus, piezoelectric crystals may be used to transmit and to receive ultrasound signals. The mechanical energy is produced in the form of vibration and is proportional to the rate of polarity changed in the electric field. Thus, the frequency of sound may be controlled by varying the frequency of the electric current acting on the crystal. High frequency electric currents in the radio frequency range must be used to produce ultrasound. To attain the most efficient signal production, the crystal must vibrate at a frequency that produces the greatest intensity. This is called the resonant frequency and is determined by the type, size, and shape of the crystal. Generally, smaller transducer crystals resonate at a higher frequency. The most efficient piezoelectric crystals for

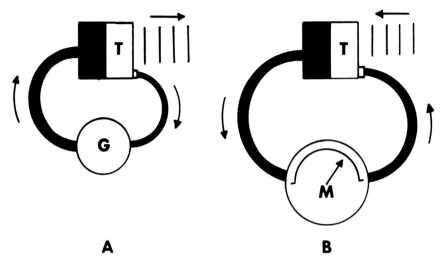

A   **B**

Fig. 1–6. Schematic illustrations of the piezoelectric effect. In *A*, an electric current generated at G is passed through a transducer crystal (T). This causes a change in the shape of the transducer, which consists of an alternating expansion and contraction of the crystal. This contraction and expansion sets up a vibration that is proportional to the frequency (number of changes in electrical polarity) of the current acting on the transducer. The vibration produces a propagating sound wave. In *B*, the process is reversed. A sound beam sets up mechanical vibrations in the transducer. These vibrations are converted to electrical energy that may be detected by a measuring device (M).

transducer use in ultrasonics are artificially constructed from lead zirconate titanate.

TYPES OF DIAGNOSTIC ULTRASOUND

Most diagnostic ultrasound today is based on reflectivity of sound waves within tissue. There are two principal types: Doppler ultrasound velocity detection and imaging reflective ultrasound.

Doppler Ultrasound Velocity Detection

Ultrasound may be used to sense motion within tissue by application of the Doppler effect principle. The Doppler effect is a change in the apparent frequency of a sound when either the source or the receiver is in motion relative to the other. If the distance is decreasing, the detected frequency is increased. If the distance is increasing, the frequency is decreased. A reflector placed in the sound beam between the source and receiver also will produce a frequency shift if it shortens or lengthens the sound-path distance between the sound source and receiver. If both the sound source and receiver are stationary, the velocity of the reflector will determine the magnitude of the frequency shift.

The cardiovascular system produces motion changes that can be measured by Doppler ultrasound velocity detectors. Two piezoelectric transducers are mounted in close proximity to each other. One transducer acts as the sound source or transmitter, and the other transducer functions as receiver. The transducers are angled slightly to detect motion in tissue deep to and between both transducers. The reflection from moving objects is due either to the pulsating vessel walls or to backscattering from the blood cells. The backscattering from the blood cells is the more important reflection. The detector discerns the frequency difference between transmitted and received signals (frequency shift) and provides this information as either an audible signal or an analog display on a monitor or recording paper. The greater the frequence shift, the greater the velocity of the blood in respect to the transmitting and receiving transducer.

Imaging Reflective Ultrasound

Imaging ultrasound employs both specular and scattered reflection. The underlying principle for all types of imaging reflective ultrasound is the same. A single piezoelectric transducer acts both as transmitter and as receiver (Fig. 1-7). To function in this manner, the transducer acts as transmitter for a short period (a fraction of a microsecond) and then converts to a receiver mode for a relatively long period. The long reception time permits a sound pulse to range out and to be reflected back to the transducer. The cycle of pulse transmissions and receptions is called the repetition rate and varies from 1000 to 8000 pulses per second. The higher repetition rates significantly limit the depth of penetration in tissue. To detect specular reflection using the same transducer for transmission and reception, the angle of beam incidence and reflection must be at or near 90°.

PRINCIPLES OF IMAGING REFLECTIVE ULTRASOUND

Imaging reflective ultrasound is based on three types of information obtained from the transmission and reception of a sound pulse: amplitude or energy intensity of the reflected signal or echo, the time duration for transmission and reflection, and the rate of change in this time duration should the cause of the echo be in motion. The way this information is affected by the factors that control reflectivity and produce diminution of the sound signal is important to an undertanding of the interaction of ultrasound with tissue.

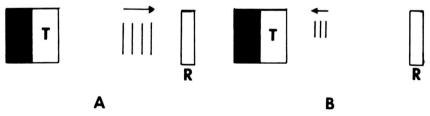

Fig. 1–7. Schematic illustrations of imaging reflective ultrasound. In *A,* a short ultrasound pulse is transmitted by the transducer (T) toward a reflector (R). In *B,* a weaker amplitude echo is reflected back to the transducer, which is now in a receive mode.

Amplitude Measurement

Amplitude or energy of sound can be measured relative to a standard value. Because sound energy varies greatly in intensity range, a logarithmic scale is used employing the decibel (db) as the unit.

$$db = 20 \log_{10} \frac{amplitude_1}{amplitude_2}$$

If $amplitude_1$ is twice $amplitude_2$, $db = 20 \log_{10} 2 = 20 \times 0.3 = 6$. Thus, a doubling of amplitude is a 6-db increase, whereas a 6-db decrease would represent a 50% fall-off in amplitude.

The db scale is used often in two ways. First, it is employed to indicate the amount of amplification used to increase a signal to a defined level. Second, the db scale is used to indicate the magnitude of an amplitude decrease relative to a reference value.

Time and Distance Relation

Time duration can be readily converted into distance.

$$\text{Velocity (c)} = \frac{\text{distance (d)}}{\text{time (t)}} \text{ or}$$

$$d = ct$$

If c is assumed to be constant in tissue and t is measured, d can be estimated.

Rate of Echo Distance Changes

Rate of change in the time dimension for production of echoes may be determined by noting the estimated distance changes over time (see *M-mode Imaging*, this chapter).

Reflection and Acoustic Impedance

The amount of sound reflected at the junction or interface between two media is determined by the difference between the acoustic impedance of the two media. In short, reflection is caused by a mismatch in acoustic impedance. Acoustic impedance (Z) is the product of density (ρ) and the propagation velocity of sound in that medium (c).

$$Z = \rho c$$

The amount of reflection is expressed in the following equation:

$$\text{Reflection} = \left(\frac{Z_2 - Z_1}{Z_2 + Z_1}\right)^2$$

When the acoustic impedance between two media is the same, there is no reflection of a beam directed to the interface between the media. When $Z_1 = Z_2$, the numerator of the equation is zero.

If either Z_1 or Z_2 is relatively large in respect to the other value, the reflection equation will approach unity or total reflection. This shows that the greater the difference between the acoustic impedance of two media (i.e., the greater the mismatch in acoustic impedance), the more sound that is reflected back. This relationship explains the great amount of reflection observed at liquid and gas interfaces and between soft tissue and bone.

Absorption

In all reflective ultrasonography, sound energy is not only subject to reflection but also may be absorbed by the tissue. Absorption is a transformation of sound energy into heat. This event is related to the viscosity of the media and to the frequency of the sound waves. The higher the frequency, the greater the absorption. The reason for the frequency dependence of absorption is the reversible conversion of some sound energy into potential energy. Potential energy is stored by the medium during the compressive phase of the sound pressure cycle and is restored back to sound energy during the relaxation phase of the cycle. This restoration is time dependent. Thus, if the time between compressions is short, as in higher frequency sound, restoration of potential energy back to the sound waves is reduced, and more of the potential energy is converted into heat.

Attenuation

All loss in the intensity in the sound signal as it is transmitted through tissue is termed attenuation. Attenuation is related to the distance traversed through the tissue and is the sum of the following factors:
1. Spreading of the ultrasound beam
2. Specular reflection
3. Scattering
4. Absorption

The sound beam that remains is the transmitted signal. Application of the transmitted ultrasound signal in medical diagnosis has been evaluated experimentally but is not used currently in clinical practice. Signal attenuation is measured with the db scale as a db decrease in reference to the intensity of the initial pulse transmitted.

Time-Gain Compensation

Because of the attenuation, which is related to the distance or depth of ultrasonic propagation through tissues, most instruments used in imaging reflective ultrasonography employ a time-gain compensation to amplify the most distant reflected signals in accordance to the time required for pulse transmission and echo return. In this manner, echoes that take a longer time (greater distance) to complete their outward propagation and to return, and that undergo greater attenuation, are amplified more than echoes that take less time. In instruments employing time-gain compensation, the amplitude boost given to the returning echoes provides a more realistic indicator of the echo-producing ability (echogenicity) of the reflector.

IMAGING REFLECTIVE ULTRASOUND SYSTEMS

Advances in imaging reflective systems have been rapid in the past 3 decades. In this section, only a brief survey of these developments will be presented with the greatest emphasis on the system used for operative ultrasonography.

One-Dimensional Systems

One-dimensional systems include A-mode and M-mode ultrasonography. In A-mode, the location of the interface producing the echo is displayed in a time-distance dimension as a spike on the monitor screen. The height or amplitude of the spike is related to the amount of reflected energy (Fig. 1-8).

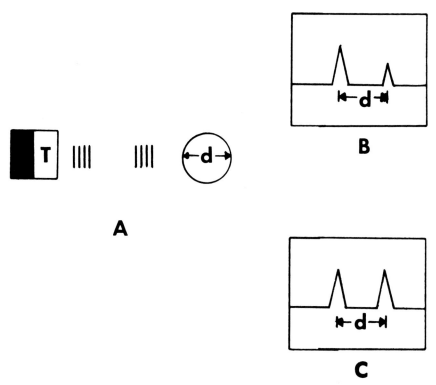

Fig. 1–8. Diagrams of A-mode. In *A*, a transducer (T) transmits a pulse toward a circular object. In *B*, the monitor display shows two amplitude spikes produced by the superficial and deep surfaces of the object. The distance (d) between the spikes corresponds to the dimension of the object. The second spike is much smaller than the first because of attenuation. In *C*, the second spike has been amplified by time-gain compensation.

Multiple spikes from multiple reflectors may be observed. Time-gain compensation is usually used to amplify the echoes from the more distant reflectors. A-mode is chiefly used to measure precisely distance and attenuation along the path of sound transmission and reflection.

In M-mode, the rate of change of a moving reflector is determined in one dimension by time-sequence recording. Time-sequence recording is similar to A-mode, except the image on the monitor screen, which is represented by a brightness dot moving on the X axis, is processed over time (Fig. 1-9). M-mode is frequently used in echocardiography to study valve and wall motion of the heart.

Two-Dimensional Systems

Two-dimensional reflective ultrasound is called B-mode imaging. The amplitude intensity owing to reflection is depicted by the brightness of a dot along a line of ultrasound transmission and reflection. The aggregation of

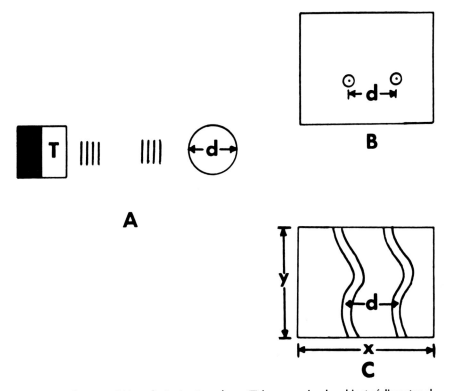

Fig. 1–9. Diagrams of M-mode. In *A,* a transducer (T) images a circular object of diameter, d, that is moving back and forth along the horizontal axis. In *B,* the monitor display at a given instant in time shows the reflection as two bright dots produced by the superficial and deep surfaces of the object. The amplitude of the reflected energy is depicted by the brightness of the dots. In *C,* the time sequence is recorded in the y axis to show the motion of dots moving in the x axis.

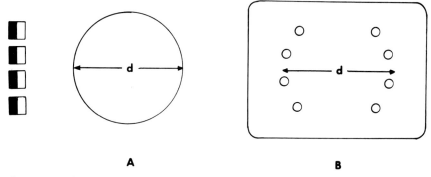

A   **B**

Fig. 1–10. Schematic illustrations of B-mode. In A, the transducer scans a circular object of diameter, d. Four transducer positions are shown. In B, the monitor shows brightness dots produced by the superficial and deep surfaces of the object for each transducer position. With multiple transducer positions, a two-dimensional image of the object can be produced in greater detail.

multiple lines composed of dots of varying brightness is used to produce a two-dimensional display (Fig. 1-10). To provide images in two dimensions, either multiple transducers must be used or a single transducer must be moved to visualize more tissue. Such motion of a transducer to extend the view through tissue is called scanning.

The tonal quality of the images produced by B-mode may be limited to show only the sharp contrast of reflectivity compared to absence of reflection. Thus, the images show bright echoes and dark areas of sonolucency. This is called bistable B-mode imaging. More often, the various shades representing different degrees of echogenicity are displayed on the monitor screen. This is termed gray-scale B-mode imaging. Two types of B-mode scanning that are based on the time duration used to develop the images are commonly used in ultrasonic diagnoses. These techniques are compound and real-time B-mode scanning.

Compound B-Mode Scanning

In compound B-mode scanning, a single transducer, which is usually hand held, is used to create a two-dimensional image on a cathode-ray tube with a persistent image capability (storage oscilloscope). The transducer establishes lines across the monitor, and the image is built up by successive development of lines. The transducer is connected to the detector by means of an articulated arm, which permits electronic sensors to track the position of the transducer (Fig. 1-11).

This type of instrumentation permits a complete composition of a tissue section by the cumulative image produced by the transducer scan. This has provided useful information in ophthalmic, abdominal, and retroperitoneal imaging. However, the development of a complete section requires a signifi-cant amount of time (usually longer than 10 seconds). Moving objects are

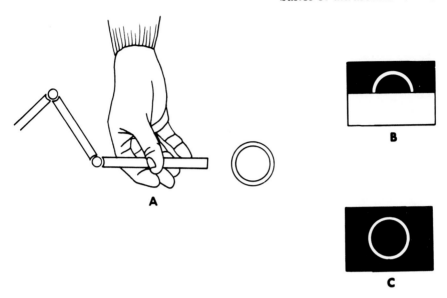

Fig. 1–11. Schematic illustrations of compound B-mode. In *A*, a transducer connected by means of an articulated arm is maneuvered by hand to scan an object. In *B*, the monitor display stores the image. About half of the image has been developed. In *C*, the entire image is shown.

displayed in terms of an average projection. Furthermore, hand-held transducer scanning introduces an element of subjectivity because of the tendency to over- or underdevelop portions of the section. These problems are reduced with real-time imaging.

Real-Time B-Mode Scanning

Real-time imaging is used in operative ultrasonography. In real-time B-mode scanning, an entire ultrasonic section is provided automatically in near-instant time. This is achieved by a battery of transducers arranged in a linear array or by means of an automatic sector scan. A sector scan is obtained by moving the transducer through an angle to image a tissue section. An imaged sector is pie shaped, and the apex is at the site of transducer placement. Automatic sector scanning is performed by motor-driven transducers or mirrors, which provide mechanical scanning, or by means of phased-array transducers, which electronically cause an ultrasound beam to sweep a sector. We have used mechanical sector-scanning transducers in operative ultrasonography (see Chap. 2). Each real-time section is a rapid buildup of scanning lines, which is displayed on a monitor screen with slight persistence of the image. Each section constitutes a frame. Frames may be changed as many as 30 times per second, thereby providing a rapidly changing sequence of views. This rapid sequence, in a practical sense, presents real-time motion (Fig. 1-12).

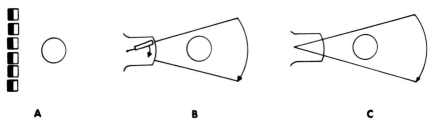

A   **B**   **C**

Fig. 1–12. Schematic illustrations of types of transducer scans in real-time B-mode. In *A,* a battery of transducers is arranged in linear array. Each transducer transmits and receives its own pulse. To achieve this with multiple transducers, the transmission of pulses for each transducer occurs at slightly different times. In *B,* a mechanical sector sweep is achieved by a transducer that moves through an angle. The transducer is automatically driven by a motor. In *C,* a phased-array transducer provides an electronic sector scan. The entire development of an image requires only a fraction of a second for each type of transducer scan.

Two types of motion observations are possible with real-time B-mode imaging: tissue motion and scanning motion. Tissue motion is intrinsic movement within the tissues. Thus, the pulsation of structures in cadence with the heartbeat or movement in phase with respirations may be seen. This type of motion is of great importance in identifying arteries and veins and helps to orient structures within a section. Scanning motion is provided by the manual movement of a transducer that is producing a real-time image. This movement is a panning action similar to cinephotography and permits the observer to obtain a panoramic view of a continuously changing section of tissue. Because of the continuity of the changing display, the observer may quickly make multiple adjustments in probe position to best view the areas of interest. This provides useful information by relating the location of different structures and by permitting a multidimensional view of key structures.

Real-time B-mode scanning is greatly facilitated by a more flexible connection between the transducer housing or probe and the detecting and display system. In compound B-mode scanning, the transducer is attached to an articulated arm, which permits electronic tracking of the transducer position. Such articular arms, because of their bulk and limited maneuverability, would be awkward to use in a sterile field during a surgical operation. Because this type of positional information is not necessary in real-time imaging, only a flexible coaxial cable is needed to connect the probe to the monitor (Fig. 1-13). This has simplified transducer-probe manipulation and is particularly important in operative ultrasonography.

CHARACTERISTICS OF ULTRASOUND IMAGES

The characteristics of the image provided by real-time B-mode scanning result from the fact that image information is obtained by the reflection rather than by the transmission of energy. This difference makes reflective

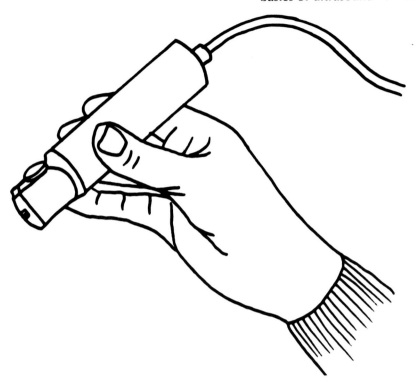

Fig. 1–13. Schematic illustration of a flexible connection between the probe containing the scanning transducer and the remainder of the ultrasound instrument. Coaxial cable is used.

images more difficult to interpret. Consequently, the distinction between transmission and reflective images must be clearly understood by the surgeon who interprets operative ultrasound images.

Geometry of Transmission and Reflective Imaging

The most familiar type of imaging information in medical diagnosis is obtained by transmission techniques using x rays. This technique involves a radiation source that sends energy through tissue and onto photographic film or an imaging monitor. The image provided is a two-dimensional display of photodensities that delineate structures as a result of the passage and attenuation of the energy. In transmission imaging, information is interpreted from a display of a projection onto a plane. In this type of imaging, two lateral dimensions are presented: height and width.

Reflective imaging in two dimensions displays only one of the two lateral dimensions, plus range. The structures that are reflective are depicted by echoes that appear on the side nearest to the transducer (Fig. 1-14). Range is the depth dimension determined by the site of placement and angulation of

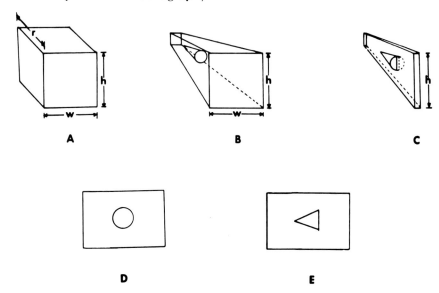

Fig. 1–14. Schematic presentations of transmission and reflective imaging. In *A,* the three space dimensions of height, width, and range are represented by h, w, and r. In *B,* transmission imaging is shown as a projection from an energy source onto a plane defined by h and w. A cone with its apex directed toward the energy source is placed as an object in the energy projection path and is imaged on the plane defined by h and w. In *C,* reflective imaging is shown as a section originating from an energy source and in the plane defined by r and h. A cone with its apex directed toward the energy source is sectioned by the plane. In *D,* the monitor display shows the transmission image. The cone appears as a circle. In *E,* the monitor display shows the reflective image. The cone appears as a triangle.

the transducer. Since the range dimension passes or "cuts" through the tissue, the reflective image display in two dimensions is a section or slice instead of a projected image. This section may be developed in any plane that is scanned by the ultrasound beam. The view of the section is oriented by the known location of the scanning transducer in respect to identified structures in the section. Size estimates can be related to structures and to the placement site of the transducer.

Transducer Function

Piezoelectric ultrasound transducers produce signals with beam dimensions that are affected by the type, shape, and size of the crystal and by the frequency of transmission.

As previously mentioned, frequency is important in determining divergence or spreading of the beam (see *Directionality,* this chapter). The beam tends to remain narrower with higher frequencies. With the high frequencies of the ultrasound range, beam width is also affected by certain characteristics of the transducers. The spread of the beam generated by an ultrasound transducer consists of a near and far field. The near field is the narrow portion of the beam. The far field is the outward spreading of the beam. With circular transducers, the distance to the junction of the near and far fields is determined by the following approximate relation:

$$D = \frac{R^2}{\lambda}$$

D is the distance to the field junction, R is the radius of the transducer, and λ is the wavelength of the ultrasound. Thus, with higher frequencies (shorter (λ), the junction is extended, and the beam retains a narrower width for a greater distance (Fig. 1-15).

Another important way to keep the beam cross section small is by using focused transducers. Focusing is provided by coupling an acoustic lens with

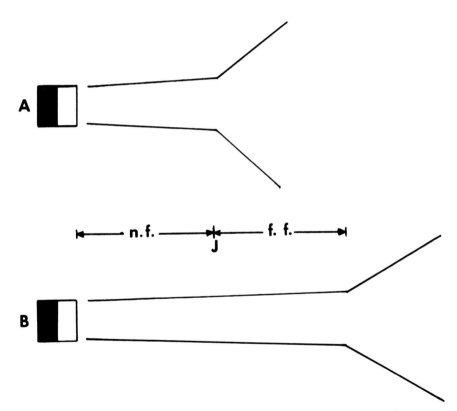

Fig. 1–15. Diagrams of beam spread. In A, the spread of the ultrasound beam is shown as a narrow near field (n.f.) and a more divergent far field (f.f.). J indicates the junction between the near and far fields. In B, the transducer produces an ultrasound beam of higher frequency than that in A. This higher frequency extends the junction between the fields farther from the transducer. A longer near field is produced, thereby resulting in an ultrasound beam that remains narrower for a longer distance.

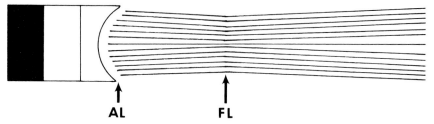

Fig. 1–16. Diagram of a focused transducer. An acoustic lens (AL) focuses the beam to narrow the cross section at a distance (the focal length [FL]) from the transducer.

the transducer surface to refract and converge the sound beams (Fig. 1-16). The focal length is the location of the narrowest beam cross section. Objects at this distance in the sound beam produce the sharpest reflective images. For this reason, the most critical portion of the image is ideally placed at the focal length. This placement can often be done by choice of probe position and by the use of acoustic windows. Unlike light, sound beams often do not have sharp focal lengths. The region of best focus may extend for a centimeter or more. In these circumstances, a focal range provides a more accurate description of the distances from the transducer that produce the clearest images (see Chap. 2, *Orientation and Interpretation,* and Chap. 3, *Transducer Probe Placement*).

Beam width or cross section affects sharpness because it determines lateral resolution. There are two types of resolution in a three-dimensional space: lateral and axial. Lateral resolution is the ability of the ultrasound scan to distinguish the separateness of two reflecting points situated on a plane at right angles to the direction of the ultrasound beam. Axial resolution is the ability to distinguish two points on the axis of the ultrasound beam (Fig. 1-17).

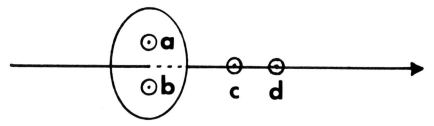

Fig. 1–17. Illustration defining lateral and axial resolution. The horizontal line is the axis of the sound beam, which is shown to intersect a circular plane at a right angle. Points a and b are on the right-angle plane. Points c and d are along the beam or transducer axis. Lateral resolution is the closest distance between points a and b that permits a distinct separation. Axial resolution is the closest distance between points c and d that permits them to be discerned separately.

Lateral Resolution

The reason why beam width determines lateral resolution can be explained by considering how echoes from points at the same range are imaged in B-mode sector scanning (Fig. 1-18). If reflection occurs from a given point along the ultrasound beam axis, the echo will be displayed on the monitor regardless of its size. If two reflecting points are located side by side at the same distance on the ultrasound beam axis and are within the same beam width, they will be interpreted as a single echo. For two

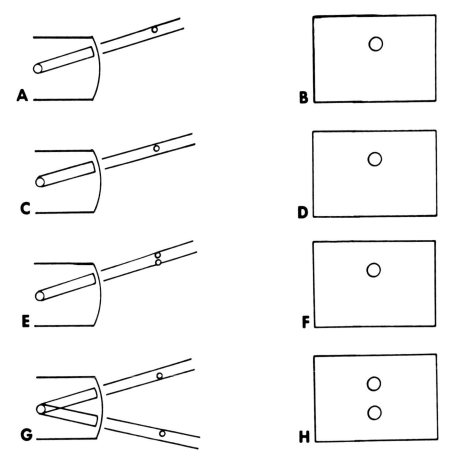

Fig. 1–18. Schematic illustrations of lateral resolution. In *A*, a point near the upper limit of the beam width is imaged on the monitor (*B*). In *C*, a point near the lower limit of the same beam as in *A* appears at the same location on the monitor screen (*D*) as in *B*. In *E*, two points are within the same beam width at the same range distance on the beam axis. In *F*, they appear on the monitor as a single point. In *G*, two points at the same range distance but more than one beam width apart are seen on the monitor (*H*) as two distinct points.

reflective points to be distinguished as two distinct echoes in the same sector scan, they must be separated by at least one beam width. In this way, narrow beam width produces higher lateral resolution.

Axial Resolution

Axial or range resolution is determined by the frequency of the ultrasound signal. The reason for this relates to the time duration of the ultrasonic pulse. If two reflective points are located at different distances on the same ultrasound beam axis, their echoes cannot be separated as two distinct echoes unless their distance apart is greater than the beam path length traversed by the moving ultrasound pulse. This is determined by both the propagation velocity of the sound and the pulse duration. The propagation velocity in tissue is essentially constant. The pulse may be varied but must consist of at least one complete sound cycle, which consists of three crossings of the zero amplitude line by the sound wave. As the frequency of the sound increases (as λ becomes shorter), the duration of the pulse may decrease and still contain the minimal number of zero crossings. Thus, the higher the frequency, the greater the axial resolution (Fig. 1-19).

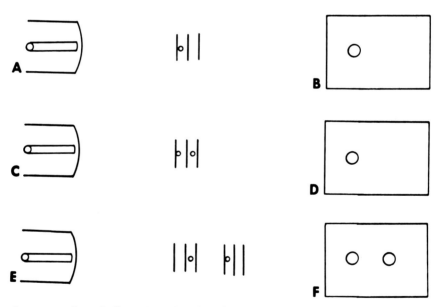

Fig. 1–19. Schematic illustrations of axial resolution. In *A*, a point in the beam axis is displayed on the monitor (*B*). In *C*, the distance between two points in the beam axis is less than the length of the ultrasound pulse. In *D*, they appear on the monitor as one point. In *E*, the distance between two points in the beam axis is greater than the length of the ultrasound pulse. In *F*, they appear as two distinct points. Since pulse length determines axial resolution and since higher frequency permits shorter pulse length, higher frequency results in greater axial resolution.

Relation of Resolution and Real-Time to Depth of Penetration

Higher-frequency ultrasound leads to higher lateral and axial resolution. However, higher frequency limits ultrasonic depth of penetration. As discussed previously (see *Absorption,* this chapter), higher-frequency ultrasound is associated with greater tissue absorption of the signal. Thus, there is a balance or trade-off in the use of ultrasound B-mode scanners that must be considered in terms of diagnostic application. When depth of penetration is necessary (e.g., whole-body scanning), the frequency must be sufficiently low to permit the required ranging. Here, resolution is compromised and may be 5 mm or more, which is still satisfactory for many diagnostic determinations. When depth of penetration need be only 3 to 4 cm, high-resolution real-time scanners employing frequencies of 7.5 to 10 MHz may be used to provide lateral and axial resolution of less than 1 mm.

Another factor limiting the depth of penetration relates to real-time imaging. To provide the best real-time imaging, the individual frames must contain maximal information and must be changed as rapidly as possible. This requires multiple pulse echoes which, in turn, require a high pulse repetition rate. At a pulse repetition rate of 8000 per second, it is only possible to range to a depth of about 6 cm because of the relatively short time available for pulses to be transmitted and returned to the transducer.

Operative ultrasonography has the advantage of not requiring great depth of penetration by ultrasonic beams. There is no need to traverse the body wall, and scanning can be performed with beam path lengths of only a few centimeters. Thus, operative ultrasound can take advantage of both high frequency for better resolution and real-time imaging with rapid pulse repetition rates. These provide images that achieve maximum sharpness and content information.

CHAPTER **2**
INSTRUMENTATION

The ultrasound equipment used in operative ultrasonography must provide useful information and meet the unique requirements of a surgical operation. To be useful at surgery, the images must be of high quality and must be obtained in a safe, simple, and rapid manner. These various requirements can be provided by recently developed, high-frequency, real-time B-mode ultrasound scanning. In this chapter, the features of ultrasound equipment especially fitted for operative application are presented, the safety of ultrasound is discussed, the operation of the instrumentation is described, and the ways ultrasonic images may be oriented and interpreted in operative imaging are considered.

The equipment for real-time B-mode ultrasonography, in terms of operator usage, consists of two major components: the transducers and the pulse processing system. These components are separate and distinct entities that are connected by a coaxial cable.

TRANSDUCERS

We have used mechanical sector-scanning transducers for operative ultrasound real-time imaging. Such transducers can be sufficiently small and are less costly to employ than are linear-array or phased-array transducers. The transducer, the motor drive, and the surrounding housing constitute the transducer-probe. We have used probes of stainless steel construction that have a window covered by a thin plastic membrane to permit passage of the sound beams.

The interior of the probe housing must be fluid tight because of the need to provide complete fluid coupling without air bubbles between the transducer and the tissue. Ultrasound is poorly transmitted through a gaseous medium, and gas-filled interfaces have a major acoustic impedance mismatch. The probe compartment immediately surrounding the moving transducer is filled with water to achieve the required fluid coupling.

Most transducers used for shallow depth (less than 6 centimeters' penetration) are designed to provide maximum lateral resolution. This is achieved by employing acoustic lenses to focus the transducer and to maintain a small transducer diameter. We have used transducers operating at 7.5 and 10 MHz that were 6 mm in diameter. The 7.5 MHz transducer is focused at 20 mm and the 10 MHz transducer at 15 mm.

The transducer-probes that we have used in operative ultrasonography have been front viewing with a sector angle of 18°. In the future, operative ultrasonography probably will be performed with side-viewing transducer-probes as well as front-viewing instruments. The availability of both instruments should provide greater flexibility in operative imaging and make possible better access to hard-to-reach areas in the operative field.

THE PULSE PROCESSING SYSTEM

The pulse processing system is the main component of the ultrasound instrument to which the transducer is connected. It has the following functions:

1. Production of a high-frequency and high-voltage electric current of short duration, which is delivered to the transducer crystal to create short-duration ultrasound pulses.

2. Reception of weak electrical signals from the transducer produced by returning sound echoes.

3. Amplification of received signals with an option to use automatic time-gain compensation.

4. Display of amplified signals in 2 dimensions with an appropriate frame change rate (20 to 30 frames per second).

5. Capability for recording and measuring images.

The pulse processing system consists of a high-voltage generator, amplifiers, filters to reduce noise, timers to measure intervals precisely, and display monitors. The system is conveniently stored within a relatively small cabinet that can be placed on a cart for portability. The high-frequency systems used for shallow penetration are generically called "small parts" scanners. Originally, they were developed for use in ophthalmology. More recently, they have been developed specifically for such other purposes as imaging of blood vessels and thyroid, parathyroid, breast, and testicular tissue.

For high-frequency shallow scanning, the transducers can be small and lower voltage generation from the pulse processing systems is sufficient. This has permitted the miniaturization of equipment, which has made small parts scanning relatively simple to operate. These features provide important practical advantages for using imaging ultrasonography in the operating room.

The display monitors used in real-time imaging employ the cathode-ray-tube principle. Two types of display monitors may be used: conventional cathode-ray oscilloscopes and television monitors, which are modified cathode-ray tubes.

A conventional cathode-ray oscilloscope consists of an electron-emitting cathode and accelerating anodes, which constitute the electron gun and place an electron beam on an imaging fluorescent screen. By means of horizontal and vertical deflectors, the electron beam that appears as a brightness spot may be made to display images. With appropriate slight persistence of the fluorescent image, the entire screen may be filled to provide complete two-dimensional frames that may be sequenced rapidly. The principal advantage of this type of electronic display is its ability to provide sharp images.

A television monitor modifies the cathode-ray tube to display automatically horizontal lines consisting of points of varying brightness. The advantages of this type of display are its ability to magnify the image and the lower cost of the video tube compared with the cost of a conventional cathode-ray oscilloscope of the same screen size. In addition, the television monitor produces bright images that can be interpreted without diminishing the operating-room lights. However, the resolution of the images of the video monitor may not be as good as the resolution of the better cathode-ray oscilloscopes.

The cathode-ray oscilloscope is primarily utilized for fine resolution imaging, particularly for precision measurements and the most faithful photographic reproductions. The television monitor is especially useful for providing enlarged images for rapid surveillance, especially if the observer is at some distance from the monitor.

The image may be photographed from the monitor screen to obtain a permanent record of a monitor display. For most clinical records, photography using quick-developing film is satisfactory, although this process reduces the gray-scale tonality in the reproduction. For the better gray-scale reproduction needed for research and teaching, conventional 35-mm photographic techniques using high-speed (400 ASA), black-and-white film is recommended. For preservation of real-time motion, videotape recording may be performed. This technique is helpful for later playback and for the selection of the best images for still photographic reproduction.

We have used two types of pulse processing systems. They differ in the dynamic range or the gray-scale quality of the display. One system is older and has a limited dynamic-range display, and the other is a more recently developed full gray-scale unit. The older system, developed by Bronson and Turner, was the first commercial B-mode real-time system used in ophthalmology.[4] To demonstrate a wide range of echo intensity, this system requires the operator to vary the sensitivity control. For a given setting, the intensity range is only 12 to 16 db which, in most instances, presents echogenic structures in a similar tone. This system employs a video monitor and is portable and simple to operate. It is easily adapted to operative ultrasonography (Fig. 2-1). The Bronson-Turner unit is manufactured by the High Stoy Technological Corporation, which also manufactures the SP-100-B model gray-scale system with a 25- to 32-db intensity range employing a cathode-ray oscilloscope (Fig. 2-2).

The limited dynamic-range system provides satisfactory images for high contrast differentiation. For example, in detecting biliary and renal calculi and in discerning fluid-filled spaces, this type of system works quite well. It is less costly and simpler to use and interpret than a more complete gray-scale system. The main advantage of the greater dynamic range of the SP-100-B model is its ability to detect more subtle changes in tissue echogenicity. This can provide more information in such conditions as atheromatous plaques and tissue inflammation. The full gray-scale imaging system may be limited by reducing the tonal range of the display. This simplifies imaging when only high-contrast displays are needed. The ability to use the same system for both limited and full gray-scale imaging provides important flexibility for operative ultrasonography.

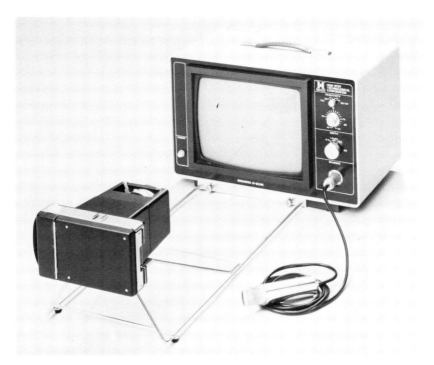

Fig. 2–1. Photo of the High Stoy Bronson-Turner ultrasound system. The display is a video monitor. The unit provides essentially bistable real-time images. (Reproduced by permission of High Stoy Technological Corp., Lake Success, NY.)

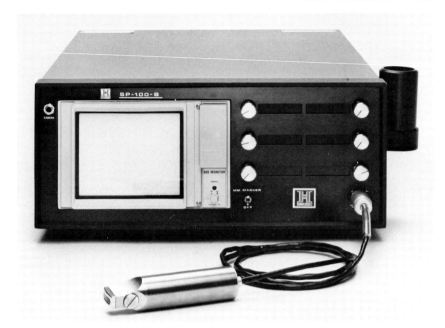

Fig. 2-2.   Photo of the High Stoy SP-100-B ultrasound system. The display is a cathode-ray oscilloscope. The unit provides gray-scale and bistable real-time images. (Reproduced by permission of High Stoy Technological Corp., Lake Success, NY.)

We have begun to use the full gray-scale imaging system with a video scan converter and television monitor. The video scan converter houses the same high-resolution oscilloscope as is contained in the pulse processing system. Images from this scope are recorded by a video camera and are displayed on a television monitor. In addition, images may be tape recorded for real-time playback. The advantage of this system is that it permits a camera to record images from the small but high-resolution cathode-ray oscilloscope and, at the same time, enables the surgeon to view a larger television monitor to interpret images during real-time scanning. This enlarged system can still be stored on a portable cart for transport and used in the operating room. Figure 2-3 is a schematic diagram of the ultrasound instrument and recording system as now used during surgical procedures.

SAFETY CONSIDERATIONS

There are two safety considerations in the use of ultrasound in the operating room. The first relates to the tissue effects of ultrasound and the second to avoidance of electrical hazards.

The principal tissue effect of ultrasound is local heating caused by absorption of energy. For most diagnostic ultrasound, this factor is negligible. For

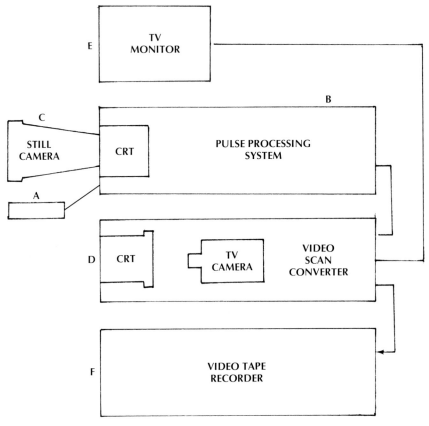

Fig. 2–3. Block diagram of the ultrasound instrument now used for operative ultrasonography. A is the transducer-probe, which connects to the pulse processing system (B). The pulse processing system contains a cathode-ray oscilloscope (CRT), which demonstrates a high-resolution ultrasound image. A still camera (C) is attached to the front of this oscilloscope. The same signal seen on the CRT of the pulse processing system is shown simultaneously on an identical CRT within the video scan converter (D). A TV camera records this image and displays it on the TV monitor. As an optional feature, the video scan converter may also transmit the signal to a video tape recorder (F).

example, in the operative ultrasonography we perform, the amount of energy applied is less than 1 milliwatt per square centimeter of contact surface (mW/cm^2). The American Institute of Ultrasound in Medicine (AIUM) has noted that no harmful biologic effects have been observed below 100 mW/cm^2. To put these values in perspective, the amount of ultrasound used in physical therapy to produce heat is about 3W/cm^2. This is 30 times the AIUM value and more than 3000 times the energy used in operative ultrasonography. At high energy levels, ultrasound produces cavitation and other deleterious tissue effects.

Ultrasound for diagnosis and therapy has been used extensively since the 1950s. It has been used widely in obstetrics to diagnose pregnancy and to measure fetal dimensions. From all these applications, no substantiated evidence has come forth regarding permanent harmful tissue effects from the medical uses of ultrasound.

The potential risk of electric devices is the inadvertent leakage of electric current to the tissue and the possibility of electric shocks or burns to the patient. Electrical safety is an important consideration in operative ultrasonography because of the decreased tolerance to electrical leakage from electric devices used inside the skin barrier. The skin provides resistance to electric current flow. Once this barrier is breached, the tissues of the body, composed mostly of electrolyte solution, provide much less resistance to electric current. For this reason, the maximum amount of current leakage permitted by hospital standards from instruments used within the body is considerably less than that permitted for devices used on the intact body surface.

Prior to usage, the entire ultrasound instrument (probe-transducer and pulse processing system) should undergo an electrical safety check similar to that used for all electric devices used in the operating room. This check should be done in addition to the safety checks provided by the manufacturer.

OPERATION OF ULTRASOUND EQUIPMENT

Before the actual surgical procedure, the operator should become familiar with how to use the ultrasound instrument. This includes some experience with preparation of the transducer-probe, use of coupling media, and familiarity with the system controls.

As mentioned previously (see *Transducers,* this chapter), the motor-driven transducer used in operative ultrasonography must be in a fluid medium that can readily transmit ultrasound. The most suitable medium is water. Saline is contraindicated because salt may enhance corrosion of internal circuitry and shorten the life span of the transducer-probe. The probe housing contains an opening for introducing and evacuating the field. The opening is kept closed by a tightly fitting screw cap.

The key factor in filling the fluid chamber surrounding the transducer is to avoid the retention of air bubbles. A 10- or 20-ml syringe is usually used to introduce the water (Fig. 2-4). During this process, the transducer-probe is gently rocked to facilitate the emergence of air bubbles. Following this step, a #18 or #19 gauge needle is fitted onto the syringe and inserted into the depths of the fluid chamber. More water is introduced through the needle to remove any bubbles that may have become trapped. After no further air bubbles emerge from the fluid chamber as a result of flushing, the opening is closed securely with the screw cap. The probe is then turned upward to permit the detection of any remaining bubbles through the plastic window. If any air bubbles are seen, the screw cap is removed and flushing with a syringe and needle is repeated. If no air bubbles are observed, the transducer-probe is ready for use.

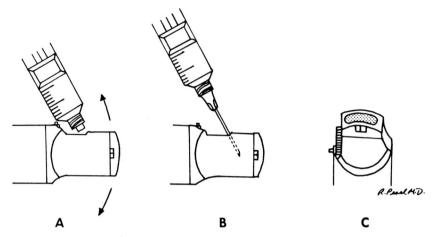

A   **B**   **C**

Fig. 2–4.   Diagrams of steps for introducing water into the probe. *A,* Water is injected through an opening in the probe housing. A 10- or 20-ml syringe is used. During this process, the transducer probe is gently rocked to facilitate the removal of air bubbles. *B,* Water is injected through a needle to make sure that all air bubbles have been removed. *C,* The transducer-probe is turned upward after replacement of the screw cap to permit an inspection for bubbles through the plastic window.

Acoustic coupling between the transducer-probe window and the tissue is a simple but essential detail that must be performed properly. As a fluid medium is needed between the transducer and the plastic window inside the probe housing, a fluid medium is also necessary between the plastic window and the tissue to be examined. As with the fluid surrounding the transducer, the fluid coupling and probe window with the tissue should be as free of gas bubbles as possible.

Two types of substances may be used to provide acoustic coupling: methylcellulose gel and saline. Methylcellulose is an inert substance that creates a viscous gel. This substance is frequently used in routine transcutaneous ultrasonography. The advantage of methylcellulose gel is its tendency to remain in place. We have found, however, that methylcellulose is not necessary for operative ultrasonography because saline works quite well. The areas of interest can usually be immersed in a saline pool. Theoretically, saline is the least-irritating fluid for contact with tissue and is always available and easy to use as a coupling media.

The controls for the pulse processing system vary according to the make and model of the ultrasound instrument used. Four basic controls may be provided. Two may be under manual control or may be automatic. These controls are the strength or intensity of the transmitted pulse and the time-gain compensation. The setting for the pulse intensity control is usually specified in the instruction manual for different types of examinations and is usually set and left undisturbed for the entire examination. The time-gain compensation control usually should be turned on to maximize reception of the deeper echoes.

Two controls are always present in high-frequency, real-time, small parts, B-mode ultrasound scanners: range setting and sensitivity.

The range setting establishes the tissue depth from which echoes are obtained. In small parts scanning, this setting is usually 0 to 6.0 cm. For transducers operating at 7.5 to 10 MHz and with a repetition rate of 8000 pulses per second used for motor-driven, automatically sweeping transducers, the maximum effective depth of tissue penetration is 6.0 cm. This has proved to be quite adequate for operative ultrasonography, and most operative examinations are performed at a range setting of 3 to 4 cm.

The sensitivity setting determines how much the weak echoes received from the tissue are amplified. The amount of amplification is measured in decibels (see Chap. 1, *Amplitude Measurement*). Usually some amplification is provided automatically. A control dial enables the examiner to increase the amplification further. Generally, it is desirable to start an examination at 10 to 20 db below maximum amplification. Too little amplification may not reveal echoes from important structures. Too much sensitivity may inordinately highlight unimportant echoes and obscure the appearance of relevant structures. Thus, a compromise setting usually has to be developed by trial. Once established for a particular type of examination, the sensitivity can often be preset and left undisturbed.

Small parts B-mode ultrasound scanners may have additional features and controls. These include the ability to magnify the image. This, in essence, permits the operator to "zoom" the image for a better view of detail. Usually, a range marker is provided that may be superimposed on the monitor screen by a control switch. This permits a more precise estimation of distances and the dimensions of structures.

ORIENTATION AND INTERPRETATION OF THE ULTRASOUND IMAGE

After the examiner has become acquainted with the operation of the ultrasound equipment, but before the equipment is used during a surgical procedure, it is important to know how images are oriented on the monitor and how they should be interpreted.

A practical way to acquire this information and gain preliminary experience with imaging ultrasound is to perform a few simple experiments using a water tank. The water tank can be any receptacle with a flat bottom that is wide enough to admit the transducer-probe and the examiner's hand. The container should be filled with water to a depth of 8 to 10 centimeters.

Angulation and Ranging Experiments

The first experiment to be described is intended to relate transducer-probe positions to the monitor image. The transducer-probe is immersed beneath the surface of the water and positioned at a right angle to the bottom of the container (Fig. 2-5, *A*). The monitor view (Fig. 2-5, *B*) shows the bottom of the container as a vertical line on the screen. The transducer-probe should

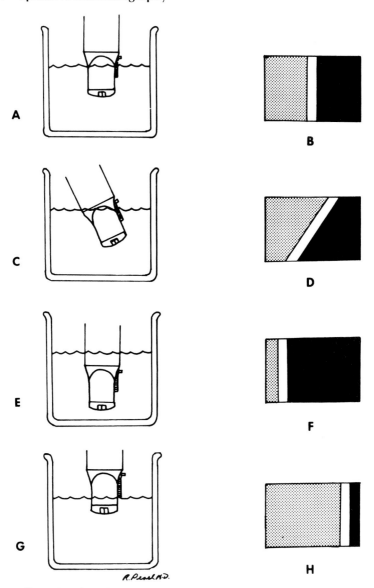

Fig. 2–5. Illustration of angulation (*A, B, C,* and *D*) and ranging (*E, F, G,* and *H*) experiments.

then be tilted to change the angle to a measurement other than 90° (Fig. 2-5, *C*). The monitor view (Fig. 2-5, *D*) shows the line produced by the echoes reflecting from the bottom of the container as slanted instead of vertical. The transducer should be returned to a right angle again. A vertical line will reappear on the monitor to represent the container bottom. The depth of the transducer probe should now be changed to bring the probe window closer and farther from the bottom of the container. This action will change the position of the vertical line depicting the container bottom. As the distance between the transducer-probe and bottom decreases (Fig. 2-5, E), the vertical lines moves closer to the left (Fig. 2-5, F). As the distance between the transducer-probe and the container bottom lengthens (Fig. 2-5, G), the vertical line moves away from the left boundary of the monitor (Fig. 2-5, H). These manipulations demonstrate the motion of a reflective surface as its distance or range is varied.

In summary, the various manipulations show that the position of the transducer-probe window is represented at the left boundary of the monitor screen. The ultrasonic image is arranged from left to right in reference to the transducer-probe position. Objects that are superficial or closer to the transducer are nearer to the left boundary of the monitor, whereas objects that are deeper or farther from the transducer are a greater distance from the left boundary of the monitor. If the transducer-probe images a straight surface at a right angle to that surface, the echoes from the surface will depict a straight vertical line. If the transducer-probe images a straight surface at an acute or obtuse angle, the line will be slanted instead of vertical. Distances between the transducer-probe and the reflective surface are represented by distances along the horizontal axis from the left boundary of the monitor screen to the echoes produced by the reflective surface.

Echogenicity and Acoustic Shadow Experiment

The purpose of this experiment is to demonstrate two key features of reflective ultrasound imaging: echogenicity and acoustic shadowing. The experiment should be performed with a hemostat placed in the ultrasound path in a water bath. The hemostat should be closed, and an image cross section should be obtained through the blade portion (Fig. 2-6, A). The cross section appears as a reflective spot to the left of the vertical line representing the container bottom (Fig. 2-6, B). The spot is bright on the aspect facing the

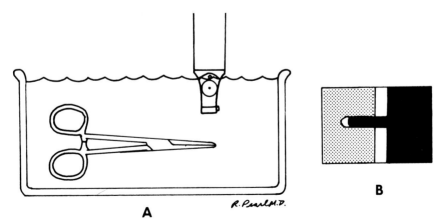

A   B

R. Pearl M.D.

Fig. 2–6. Illustrations of the echogenicity and acoustic shadow experiment.

left boundary of the monitor. Immediately to the right of this zone of brightness, the spot is dark, and this area of darkness passes straight back to the extreme right margin of the monitor screen.

The zone of brightness depicts the highly reflective surface of the hemostat. This structure is considered highly echogenic. A measure of the high degree of echogenicity is the extreme brightness of the surface echoes. A more quantitative measure of the extreme echogenicity is the persistence of the surface echoes from the steel hemostat after the sensitivity is turned down to or near its lower limit.

The dark area starting at the bright spot and passing to the extreme right of the image screen is the acoustic shadow produced by the highly reflective object. This occurrence is similar to a shadow produced by light. The acoustic shadow passes behind the object producing the shadow. The more reflective the object, the denser the shadow. With steel, the reflection is total; consequently, a prominent shadow is cast. If a second reflective object is in the acoustic shadow, it may not be detected because there is insufficient sound energy to produce an image. In the illustration, the acoustic shadow produced by the hemostat cuts through and obscures a small portion of the reflective container's bottom surface.

Superior-Inferior Orientation Experiment

Motion in a lateral dimension is depicted in this experiment by moving the hemostat parallel to the surface of the transducer-probe window (Fig. 2-7, A). The hemostat image on the monitor screen is observed to move in an up-and-down direction as the hemostat is passed back and forth in front of the transducer (Fig. 2-7, B). With a few such maneuvers, one can determine which portion of the transducer-probe window is associated with the superior aspect or "top" of the sector field and which is associated with the inferior or "bottom" of the field as shown on the monitor screen. This

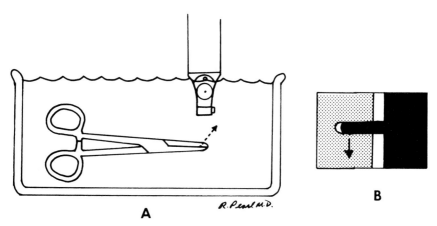

A   R. Pearl M.D.   **B**

Fig. 2–7. Illustration of the superior-inferior orientation experiment.

orientation should be known for each transducer and noted by some identifying marker on the surface of the probe (e.g., the screw cap).

If the orientation is not known for a transducer about to be used during a
surgical procedure, this simple experiment may be performed to obtain this
information.

Lateral Resolution Experiment

This experiment shows the limits of lateral resolution of the ultrasound
instrument. The hemostat should be opened and the prongs spread about 1
millimeter apart at their tips (Fig. 2-8, A). The open hemostat should be
rotated to permit each prong and the gap between them to be imaged in
cross section. If the open hemostat now appears as two discernible spots
(Fig. 2-8, B), the lateral resolution of the ultrasound instrument is at least 1
millimeter. By slowly opening and shutting the hemostat and noting the
distance between the prongs, the actual lateral resolution may be estimated.

Focal Distance Experiment

In this experiment, optimal discrimination produced by imaging in the
focal range is demonstrated. A transducer focused at 15 and 20 mm should
be used. With the transducer submerged in the water bath, the tip of the
closed hemostat is moved along the beam axis. The reflective spot is smaller
and brighter at the focal distance than at any other location along the path.
The focal distance is the ideal distance for imaging (Fig. 2-9).

In tissue imaging, an attempt should be made to place the area of greatest
interest near the focal distance of the transducer. In operative ultrasonography, the area of greatest interest may be only a centimeter or less beneath
the surface (e.g., lumen of a common bile duct or artery). In these situations,
the examination is best performed through a layer of saline. By maintaining
a distance of 5 to 10 mm in the coupling fluid superficial to the surface of a

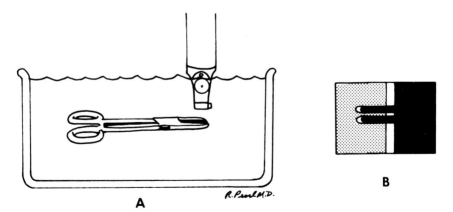

A   R. Prul M.D.   **B**

Fig. 2–8.   Illustration of the lateral resolution experiment.

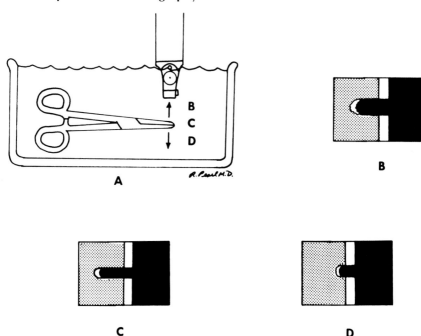

Fig. 2–9. Illustration of the focal distance experiment. *A,* A hemostat is moved along the beam axis. Three positions along this axis are marked to indicate a point at less than the focal distance (*B*), a point at the focal distance (*C*), and a point beyond the focal distance (*D*). In *B,* *C,* and *D,* the respective monitor images are seen. The image of the hemostat cross section in *C* is sharper and smaller than in *B* or *D.*

common duct or artery, the area of greatest interest is placed closer to the focal distance of the transducer. Furthermore, the superficial aspect of the structure can be more clearly visualized. The coupling fluid used to place the transducer at a greater distance from the object is called an acoustic window. Acoustic windows are used frequently in operative ultrasonography because of the superficial presentation of many organs and tissues in the operative field.

CHAPTER **3**
GENERAL
TECHNIQUES

Before considering the specific uses of ultrasonography in various types of operations, this chapter reviews some general techniques that apply to most of operative ultrasonography. This review includes a description of how to prepare a sterile transducer-probe for operative ultrasonography and how the ultrasound instrumentation (transducer-probe and pulse processing system) is best deployed in the operative field. The general principles to be used in the technique for proper placement of a transducer-probe are presented in detail. Finally, the basic maneuvers employed in operative tissue scanning are reviewed in terms both of the types of manipulations performed and the resulting images produced by these manipulations.

TRANSDUCER-PROBE STERILITY

There are two methods for providing a sterile transducer-probe: cold gas sterilization or use of a disposable plastic sterile cover.

Cold Gas Sterilization

The cleaned transducer-probe is emptied of all coupling fluid in the chamber around the transducer. The screw cap is put into place and rotated just enough to fix it in place but is kept loose enough to permit gas to penetrate the probe interior. The transducer is then doubly wrapped. The wrapped package is then processed through an ethylene oxide gas sterilizer. Because the plastic window and the coaxial cable cannot withstand excessive heat, the temperature of any step in the sterilization process must not exceed 120° F. After the wrapped probe is sterilized, the package must be allowed to air to permit removal of the ethylene oxide in contact with the outside surface of the probe. Ethylene oxide is toxic to tissue and should be allowed to evaporate prior to contact of the sterile instrument with tissue. This process requires several days for shelf-stored items. To accelerate the removal of ethylene oxide, aeration chambers may be employed. However, some of the standard aerators used to remove ethylene oxide that we have examined function at temperatures that are too high for the transducer-probe (above 120° F). The aeration system to be used for the transducer-probe should be temperature monitored. If this temperature is above 120° F, a room temperature process should be employed. A room temperature procedure, which we have devised, may be performed in the operating room.

Rapid room temperature aeration is achieved with the use of a vacuum bottle or jar found in most operating rooms. The principle involved is to force a large volume of room air through the container to produce a rapid exchange of gas. The sterilized package containing the transducer probe is placed within the vacuum bottle, and the lid is tightly reapplied. The vacuum is turned on and room air is allowed to enter the bottle through the port to which suction tubing would normally be connected. Aeration is carried out for a period of 8 hours (Fig. 3-1).

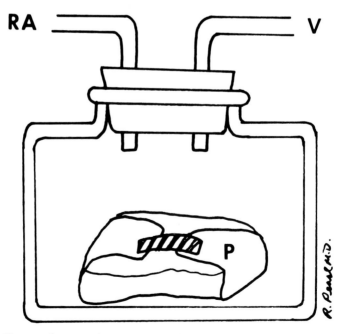

Fig. 3–1. Diagram of an operating room vacuum bottle used to hasten the aeration of a wrapped transducer-probe (P) at room temperature. Room air (RA) is allowed to enter one spout while vacuum (V) is applied to another opening. This produces a rapid air exchange, which aerates the probe in 8 hours.

When ready for use, the sterile transducer-probe is placed on the nurse's table. The transducer-probe chamber is filled with sterile water using the same technique as previously described (see Chap. 2, *Operation of Ultrasound Equipment*).

Disposable Sterile Probe Cover

The clean but nonsterile transducer-probe is filied with water and is placed within a disposable plastic sterile cover.

We have used a cover composed of a double layer of 1-mil (0.001 inch) polyethylene fused together. Single layer 1-mil polyethylene proved to contain too many pin holes to be used as a sterile barrier. Fusing two layers together has eliminated the porosity problem and has provided an inexpensive plastic cover. The probe cover is a 6-foot-long cylinder, 3 inches in diameter, and closed at one end.

The steps in covering the transducer-probe are as follows (Fig. 3-2):

1. A sterile-clad operator (surgeon or nurse) holds open the lumen of the sleeve that has been folded prior to packaging.

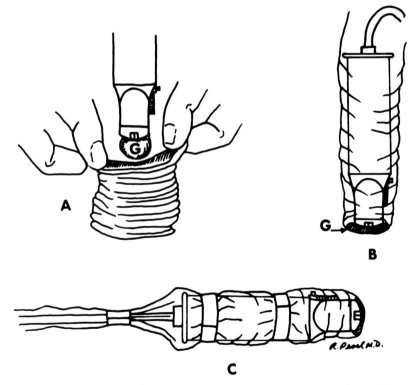

Fig. 3–2. Diagram of steps followed when covering a transducer probe with a sterile, disposable, plastic sleeve. *A,* The sterile hands of an operator hold a previously folded plastic cover. A generous amount of methylcellulose gel (G) is introduced into the closed end of the probe cover. *B,* The transducer-probe is covered by the plastic sleeve. The probe window is immersed in the methylcellulose gel. *C,* The plastic sleeve is secured with sterile adhesive tape.

2. A generous (20 to 30 ml) amount of methylcellulose gel is introduced into the closed end of the plastic sleeve.

3. The transducer-probe is inserted by the circulating nurse, and the plastic cover is brought over the coaxial cable.

4. Sterile adhesive is wrapped tightly around the plastic cover near the widow end of the transducer. This adhesive-tape wrap should insure that the methylcellulose gel is squeezed into the distal-most portion of the sleeve and is kept there by the tight wrap of the tape. Great care should be exercised so that no air bubbles are trapped in the gel between the probe window and the plastic cover. The adhesive tape should also fix the probe cover to minimize wrinkling. The seam that closes the end of the plastic sleeve should be placed along the side of the probe and not over the probe window.

5. Additional wraps of sterile adhesive tape should be placed to fix the plastic cover to the proximal portion of the probe and to the cable.

The choice of whether to obtain a sterile transducer-probe is determined largely by the frequency of usage. The time cycle for cold gas sterilization is about 12 hours with the rapid aeration procedure. This usually means that a transducer-probe may only be used once a day. Consequently, if the usage requirements for the transducer probe are once a day or less, cold gas sterilization may be used. This avoids the effort of applying a sterile cover. On the other hand, if the transducer-probe is used more than once per day, the sterile disposable cover is recommended. With experience, the sterile cover can be applied with little effort and no significant time delay.

DEPLOYMENT OF THE ULTRASOUND INSTRUMENTATION

The pulse processing system should be placed on the opposite side of operating table from the surgeon. The system should be positioned to permit the surgeon to view clearly the monitor screen across the patient. The sterile transducer-probe should be fixed to the operating field by folding a towel around the cable about 50 cm below the transducer-probe and applying two towel clips. The towel clips maintain the folded towel about the cable and anchor the cable to the drape sheet at the edge of the surgical field (Fig. 3-3).

The control settings on the pulse processing system should be adjusted. The range setting should be appropriate for the operation. Usually, this setting should be at the 3- to 4-cm level. The sensitivity setting should be positioned usually to 10 to 20 db below the maximum amplification.

During ultrasonography, an individual (technician, nurse, or physician) who has some familiarity with the ultrasound instrumentation should be available to assist the operator in the operative field. This individual connects the coaxial cable to the pulse processing system, adjusts sensitivity, and takes photographs of the monitor screen.

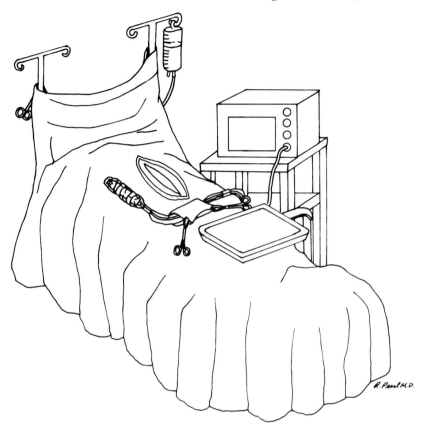

Fig. 3–3. Illustration of the deployment of the ultrasound instrumentation in the operative field. The sterile transducer-probe is fixed to the operative field by folding a towel about the cable and applying two towel clips to anchor the towel and cable to the field. The pulse processing system and monitor are on the opposite side of the patient from where the surgeon stands.

TRANSDUCER-PROBE PLACEMENT

The area to be examined by ultrasonography should be exposed to the fullest extent possible. Such exposure requires sufficient retraction to present the area of interest without interposition of other structures. The operator should keep in mind the spatial orientation of the transducer-probe in terms of the image that will appear on the monitor. In particular, the superior and inferior aspects of the sector should be relatable to the operative field. The transducer-probe is then placed over the area of interest. This initial positioning or "dry" placement is done before any saline is added.

The "dry" placement of the transducer-probe is intended to permit the operator to identify as precisely as possible anatomic landmarks and their location in reference to the transducer-probe. An important aspect of "dry" placement is knowing exactly how far the end of the probe is from the surface of the tissue. If the area of interest is likely to be deeper than 1 centimeter, the transducer-probe may be placed in direct contact with the tissue. However, if the probable area of interest is more superficial (less than 1 centimeter), the transducer should be held ½ to 1 centimeter from the surface of the tissue. It is important to find a comfortable position for hand holding the transducer-probe because a constant geometric relation between the probe and the tissue must be maintained. This can be facilitated by bracing the hand or wrist against a stable object in or near the operative field.

The operative field between the tissue and the end of the transducer-probe should be flooded with saline. The saline should be warm and introduced into the field with minimal production of bubbles. We have found that the best way to introduce a relatively large amount of saline is by decanting it from a container (Fig. 3-4). Using a syringe for this purpose more often introduces air bubbles because the fluid injection is usually more forceful.

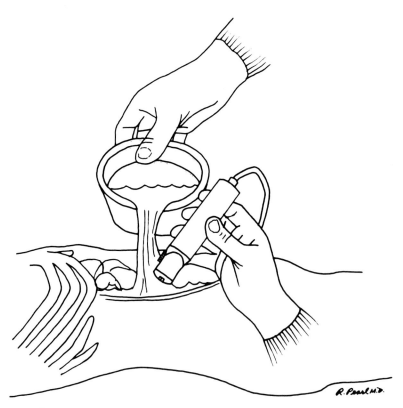

Fig. 3–4. Illustration of introduction of saline to provide acoustic coupling. While the operator holds the transducer-probe in "dry" placement over the area of interest, an assistant decants warm saline into the operative field.

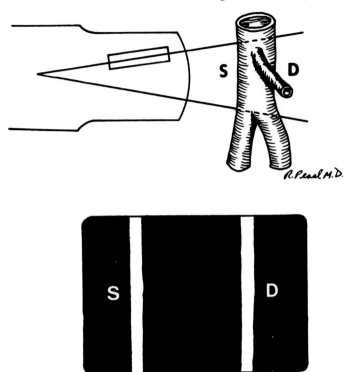

R. Pearl M.D.

Fig. 3–5. A blood vessel with a side branch is scanned from the side. The side branch is not included in the image on the monitor screen. The superficial vessel wall (S) is nearest the transducer-probe and appears closer to the left-hand border of the screen than does the deeper vessel wall (D). The transducer-probe is located at the left-hand border of the screen.

The amount of saline should be sufficient to submerge the probe window completely.

As soon as the saline has been introduced and the transducer-probe is in "wet" placement over the tissue, the monitor screen should be checked to make sure that an appropriate image is presented.

The image on the monitor must be oriented in terms of the transducer-to-object geometry. In most B-mode imaging, the transducer-probe is at the left-hand margin of the monitor screen. Thus, structures near the left border are superficial to structures farther from the left border of the monitor screen. In Figure 3-5, a blood vessel is scanned from the side, and the superficial and deep walls are shown on the monitor. In Figure 3-6, the blood vessel is scanned from a different transducer-probe location that shows a side branch on the deep surface of the blood vessel.

If the transducer-probe is held in direct contact with the tissue, the probe must not exert any undue pressure on the tissues. In particular, pressure on a pliable hollow structure may compress and distort the image sufficiently to preclude its recognition (Fig. 3-7).

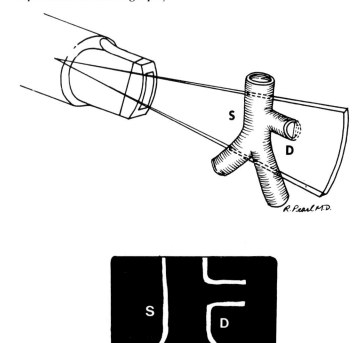

R. Pearl M.D.

Fig. 3–6. The same blood vessel that was scanned in Figure 3–5 is scanned from a different location to include the side branch. On the monitor, the side branch is seen to arise from the deeper vessel wall (D), which is at a greater distance from the left-hand border of the monitor screen than is the superficial wall (S).

If the transducer-probe is held at a slight distance from the tissue, the distinct line of the tissue surface should clearly be visible on the monitor (Fig. 3-7, *F*). The space on the monitor between its left boundary and the tissue surface is the acoustic window (see Chap. 2, *Orientation and Interpretation*). The withdrawal of the transducer-probe by a few millimeters is advisable in most examinations in which the probe is placed in contact with the tissue. This withdrawal creates an acoustic window and enables the operator to view the surface of the structure being examined. Performing this maneuver also may provide assurance that the transducer-probe has not unduly compressed the tissue.

SCANNING MANEUVERS

Once the transducer-probe is in "wet" placement and a satisfactory image has appeared on the monitor, the automatic sweeping action of the transducer produces a sector scan through the tissue. To provide additional information, the transducer should be moved by hand to create additional scanning views through the tissues. The various types of scanning maneu-

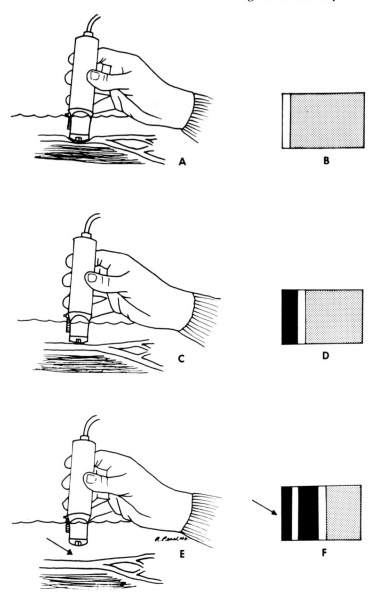

Fig. 3–7. Illustration of transducer-probe placement. *A*, A superficial, hollow, tubular structure is compressed by the probe. In *B*, the monitor view of *A* only shows an echogenic area at the extreme left side of the screen. The lumen of the structure is not discernible. *C*, The probe is in contact with the surface of a superficial, hollow, tubular structure but is not compressing the lumen. In *D*, the monitor view of *C* shows a lumen and the deep wall of the hollow structure. However, the superficial wall cannot be seen. *E*, The probe is held at a slight distance from the surface of a superficial, hollow, tubular structure. The fluid between the probe window and the tissue (arrow) provides an acoustic window. In *F*, the monitor view of *E* shows the superficial wall, lumen, and deep wall of the tubular structure. The area nearest the left boundary of the screen (arrow) is an acoustic window provided by the coupling fluid.

vers used in operative ultrasound will be described in terms of the manipulations performed. Then the resulting images produced by these maneuvers will be reviewed.

Types of Scanning Maneuvers

There are four basic scanning maneuvers commonly used with a real-time, mechanically driven transducer-probe. These basic maneuvers are often combined to produce more complex scans. Two of these maneuvers consist of angulating the probe, whereas the two other maneuvers entail moving the probe along a path.

The two angulation maneuvers are performed either within a single sector plane or to image multiple new sector planes. In both angulation maneuvers, the probe end remains in relatively stationary contact with the tissue surface or is fixed a few millimeters from the tissue surface. The angulation maneuvers are achieved by rotating the transducer probe to develop a new viewing angle. The apex of the angle is the fixed position of the probe. If the sweep of the angle is in the plane being automatically sector scanned, the maneuver is called longitudinal angulation (Fig. 3-8, A). If the sweep of the manual angulation is at a right angle to the plane being automatically scanned, the maneuver is called transverse angulation (Fig. 3-8, B).

The two scanning movements of the transducer-probe along a path may be either along the plane developed by the automatic sector scan or at a right angle to this plane. If the path is along the automatic sector plane, the maneuver is called a longitudinal scan (Fig. 3-8, C). If the probe is moved from side to side, the maneuver is called a transverse scan (Fig. 3-8, D).

As mentioned previously, the four basic scanning maneuvers are often combined. Usually during a longitudinal or transverse scan, one of the angulation maneuvers is performed simultaneously.

Images Produced by Scanning Maneuvers

Each scanning maneuver results in a different series of images. Some general considerations dictate the maneuver that is most suitable for a particular application. Some of the maneuvers cannot be employed because of tissue exposure or physical constraints at the operative sites. Each scanning image will be described and its advantages and limitations discussed to more fully explain the indications for use.

Longitudinal angulation provides an extension of the image already in view without appreciably changing the transducer-probe position (Fig. 3-9). This maneuver is helpful when an area of interest is already seen and the operator wishes to extend the field of view above or below the imaged sector. The particular advantage of this maneuver is that the field of view can be extended without losing a critical transducer-probe position. This maneuver is also helpful when the transducer-probe cannot be physically manipulated in a longitudinal scan path. The main disadvantage of this maneuver is

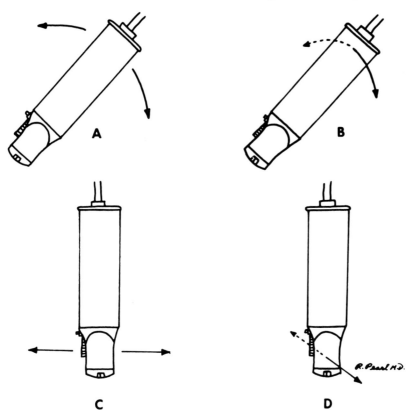

Fig. 3–8. Schematic representation of the four basic scanning maneuvers. *A,* Illustration of longitudinal angulation. *B,* Illustration of transverse angulation. *C,* Illustration of longitudinal scanning. *D,* Illustration of transverse scanning.

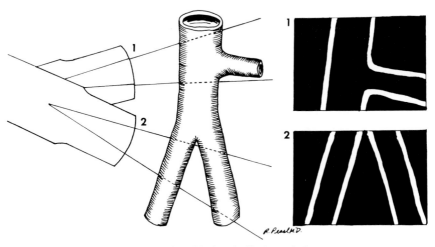

Fig. 3–9. Illustration of sectors produced by longitudinal angulation.

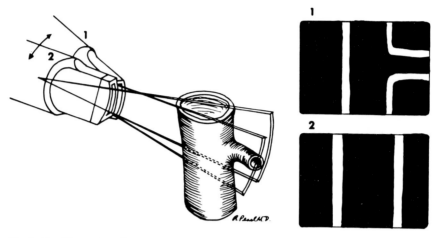

Fig. 3–10. Illustration of sectors produced by transverse angulation.

the greater range required to demonstrate the same object because more tissue is traversed with an acute angle than with a normal angle.

Transverse angulation displays multiple sections that all originate at the site of transducer-probe placement (Fig. 3-10). This maneuver is most helpful in surveying the regions immediately lateral to the main area of interest. For example, transverse angulation is used to image the mural details or luminal contents during the examinations of a hollow tubular structure. This maneuver is especially useful in combination with longitudinal scanning of a hollow viscus. In this procedure, image orientation to the main area of interest is retained while the more peripheral aspects of the lumen or the wall of the structure are checked.

Longitudinal scanning usually can be accomplished rapidly because the visualization of a continuous panoramic image requires less time for reorientation than does visualization of the totally new tissue sectors produced by transverse scanning. Longitudinal scanning shows the connection between progressive views (Fig. 3-11) that helps to maintain orientation and facilitates the recognition of structures. Longitudinal scanning requires the availability of a relatively large surface of tissue to provide the needed scan paths. Furthermore, there must be sufficient room to maneuver the transducer-probe within the depths of the operative field.

Transverse scanning can also be achieved fairly rapidly, but usually not as fast as longitudinal scanning, because the operator must be reoriented to new sectors and must relate them to previous views (Fig. 3-12). As with longitudinal scanning, transverse scanning requires relatively large tissue surfaces and enough space to manipulate the transducer-probe in the operative field.

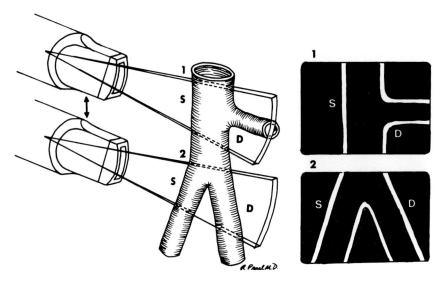

Fig. 3–11. Illustration of sectors produced by longitudinal scanning.

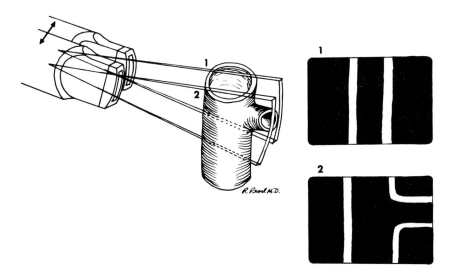

Fig. 3–12. Illustration of sectors produced by transverse scanning.

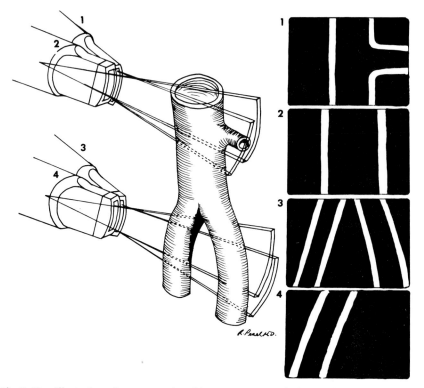

Fig. 3–13. Illustration of sectors produced by transverse angulation combined with longitudinal scanning.

Scanning maneuvers are usually combined with angulation. The most common combination is transverse angulation performed with longitudinal scanning (Fig. 3-13). This combination of maneuvers provides a rapid scan of an elongated structure (such as a blood vessel or bile duct) and, at the same time, allows each site along the course of the structure to be surveyed in different planes.

When the gallbladder is absent or cannot be found, identification of any longitudinal hollow structure to the right of the hepatic artery that could be the common duct should be pursued. This should be done in a manner that will determine the relation of the ductular structure to the duodenum by scanning toward the duodenum as far as possible. If a ductular structure is detected superior to the duodenum, scanning should be continued onto the anterior surface of the duodenum. This may trace the extension of the duct to a retroduodenal position in a course similar to that of the common duct. Once the common duct is tentatively located, aspiration with a fine bore needle may be performed to confirm the presence of bile.

Abnormally placed hepatic arteries may also be identified by ultrasound. Figure 4–2 illustrates the right hepatic artery between the common duct and the portal vein. The artery was clearly identified because of its pulsations in real-time imaging.

GALLBLADDER CONTENT ASSESSMENT

In the workup of a patient who may have biliary tract disease, a number of effective preoperative diagnostic studies are available to determine if calculi are present in the gallbladder. The most frequently used procedures are oral cholecystography, intravenous cholecystography, ultrasound, and nuclear excretory scanning. If the surgeon is uncertain about the presence of stones in the gallbladder prior to operation, palpation of the gallbladder, which is part of the initial exploration, will usually reveal stones. Problems in operative diagnosis occur when preoperative studies either are not done or are not definitive and when palpation of the gallbladder does not provide adequate information. Lack of such information may be the result of increased thickness of the gallbladder wall, a tensely distended gallbladder, adhesions to the surface of the gallbladder, or a combination of these factors.

Operative ultrasonic assessment of gallbladder content may be used in operations for suspected biliary disease or in operations for other intra-abdominal conditions in which the gallbladder should be evaluated. In either instance, the uncertainty or absence of preoperative studies in addition to inadequate information obtained from palpation presents a problem for the surgeon. If biliary disease is suspected, the surgeon usually proceeds with cholecystectomy on the basis of wall thickening or inflammation. If the operation is performed for another condition, the primary problem is usually addressed, and the surgeon must choose between deferring further investigation of the gallbladder and doing further exploration by means of tissue dissection or aspiration.

Operative ultrasonography may be useful in both of these situations. During an operation for suspected calculus cholecystitis, ultrasonography may confirm nonpalpable calculi in the gallbladder or cystic duct and indicate their size. Ultrasonography may be done early during the operation before the gallbladder is grasped with crushing clamps, which commits the surgeon to removal of the gallbladder.

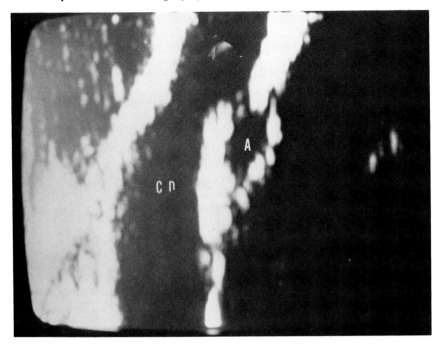

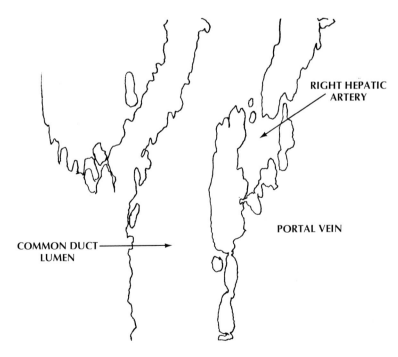

Fig. 4–2. Sonogram that shows a common duct (CD) with the right hepatic artery (A) in cross section between the duct and portal vein.

Identifying small calculi with this technique may be particularly important. The presence of small gallbladder calculi increases the likelihood of choledocholithiasis. Confirmation of small stones in the gallbladder early during the operation permits the surgeon to assess more quickly the situation and to plan the operative management.

In abdominal operation for conditions other than biliary disease, palpation of the gallbladder is the principal means of knowing whether gallbladder calculi are present. When palpation cannot provide satisfactory information about the presence of gallbladder calculi, operative ultrasonography may resolve any questions without aspiration or further dissection to remove adhesions.

Technique

If the operator has no previous operative experience with ultrasonography, a practice exercise is advisable using a freshly removed, unopened gallbladder containing calculi. This exercise is best done after the operation when the surgeon can devote full attention to practice without taking operating time.

The gallbladder specimen should be placed in a basin of saline. The transducer-probe is immersed in the saline bath, and the gallbladder wall and its contents are examined by both longitudinal and transverse scanning (Fig. 4-3). The purpose of this exercise is to obtain experience with the

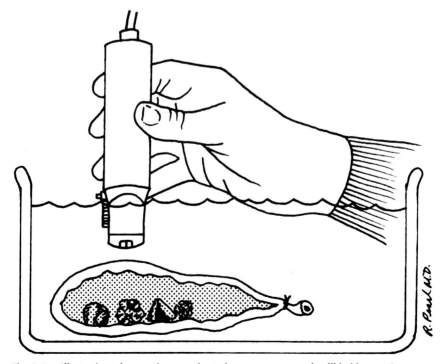

Fig. 4–3. Illustration of a practice exercise to image an unopened gallbladder specimen.

different images produced by the various transducer-probe scanning maneuvers. In addition, the appearance of the images produced by various probe placements can be better understood (Fig. 4-4). For example, the images produced by placing the transducer-probe in contact with the gallbladder may be compared with the images obtained when an acoustic window is used.

In operative ultrasonic examination of the gallbladder, the predominant maneuver is the longitudinal scan (Fig. 4-5). Transverse angulation should be performed concomitantly. These maneuvers provide the most rapid scanning of the gallbladder. When a stone is found or suspected, transverse scanning may help to demonstrate more clearly any abnormality and to provide a more systematic survey of the area of interest.

Findings

The normal gallbladder has an echogenic wall and sonolucent lumen. The principal objective of the survey is to assess the gallbladder wall and the luminal content.

The normal gallbladder wall is thin (less than 3 mm thick). Thickening of the wall is a sign of inflammation and may be detected by ultrasonography (Fig. 4-6).

An image of the gallbladder wall that is not abnormal but may be mistaken for a disorder is produced by a folded gallbladder (Fig. 4-7). In one instance, preoperative ultrasonography was interpreted as suggesting a bifid gallbladder. During the operation, ultrasonography showed a "septum" that proved to be a double layer of gallbladder wall caused by folding.

Any echogenicity within the gallbladder should be carefully evaluated as possible biliary calculi. A number of image patterns of calculi relate to their size and echogenicity. Figure 4-8 shows large echogenic calculi, whereas Figure 4-9 shows smaller calculi.

The principal features in recognizing gallbladder calculi are their echogenicity and the accompanying acoustic shadows. The echogenicity of biliary calculi is usually seen at the outer edge nearest the transducer-probe because most of the sound is reflected at or near the stone surface. Consequently, the superficial outer zone of the calculus, but not the entire stone, is demarcated. Thus, a calculus may appear as a thin crescent rather than as an image shaped more like a biliary calculus. Passing from behind the echogenic zone is the acoustic shadow. The acoustic shadow is related to the amount of sound reflected at the outer zone of the stone. Where echogenicity is high, a dense acoustic shadow is seen; where sound penetrates the stone, the acoustic shadow is less dense. The presence of these two features—an echogenic zone and an acoustic shadow—is key to the diagnosis of calculi.

The recognition of an acoustic shadow not only is useful in diagnosing the presence of stones, but also is important in avoiding a possible error in interpretation. This error may occur when several large stones are in close

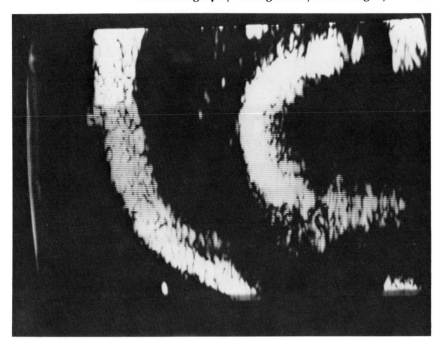

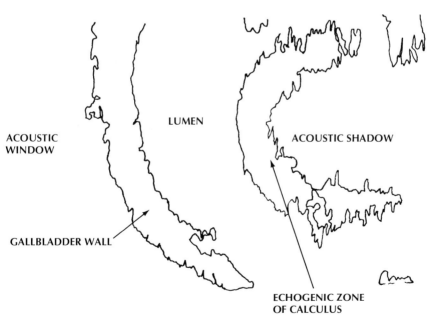

ACOUSTIC
WINDOW

LUMEN

ACOUSTIC SHADOW

GALLBLADDER WALL

ECHOGENIC ZONE
OF CALCULUS

Fig. 4–4. Sonogram of an excised gallbladder within a saline bath. The presence of an
acoustic window permits good visualization of the gallbladder wall. A large calculus with a
highly echogenic outer zone is present. An acoustic shadow is seen behind the echogenic
outer zone.

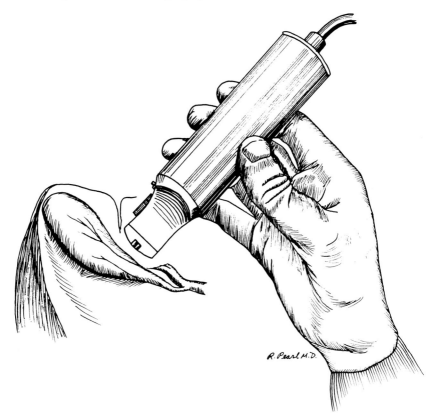

Fig. 4–5. Illustration showing longitudinal scanning of the gallbladder.

proximity to the gallbladder wall. In this situation, the echogenic zone of the calculi may not be distinguished from the echoes produced by the gallbladder wall. The acoustic shadow behind the echogenic zone may then be mistaken for a clear gallbladder lumen. This may lead to missing the stones entirely.

The best way to avoid this error is to pay attention to certain details regarding the appearance of the gallbladder wall and the echogenic zones of calculi. First, an acoustic window should be utilized in positioning the transducer-probe. This will insure that the gallbladder wall is included in the image. Merely placing the probe in contact with the gallbladder surface may cause the stone echo to be mistaken for the gallbladder wall. Second, one should look for certain distinctive echo features. One feature is the demarcation space between the wall echoes and the stone echoes. This space may not be great if the calculi are close to the wall. Another feature is a difference in echogenicity. The stone echoes are usually more echogenic and may, in this manner, be distinguished from the wall. A simple way to confirm the

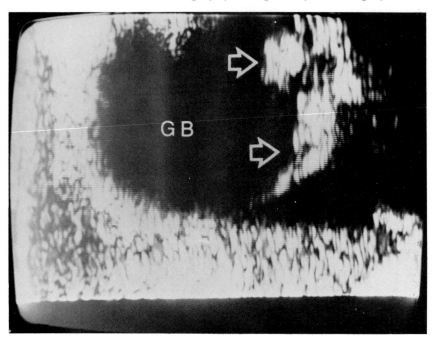

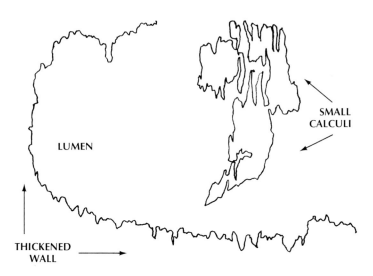

Fig. 4–6. Sonogram of gallbladder with thickened wall. Small calculi are also present but could not be palpated because of the thickened wall.

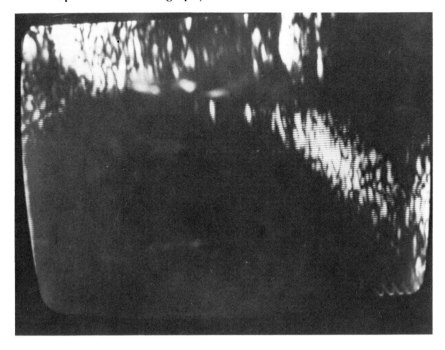

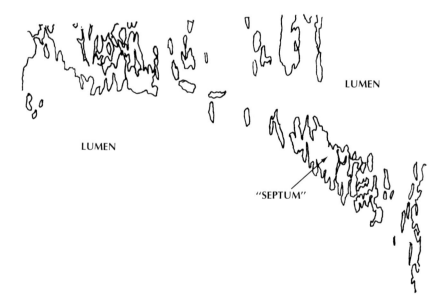

Fig. 4–7. Sonogram of a folded gallbladder. The "septum" between the two cystic cavities is a double layer of gallbladder wall.

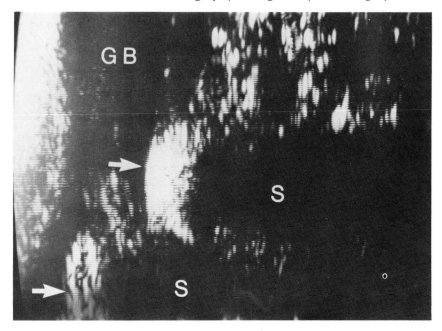

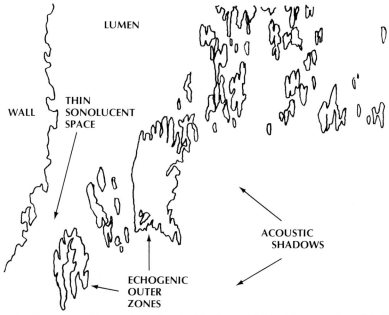

Fig. 4–8.   Sonogram of large echogenic calculi in the gallbladder (GB) near the gallbladder wall. A thin, sonolucent space can be seen between the gallbladder wall and the echogenic outer zones of the calculi. The calculi echoes are more intense than the gallbladder wall echoes. The rounded contour of the gallbladder calculi show a scalloped appearance. The calculi produce acoustic shadows (S), which pass to the extreme right margin of the sonogram.

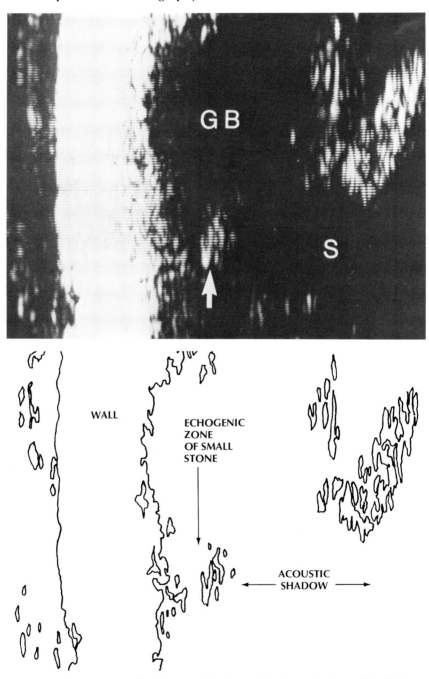

Fig. 4–9. Sonogram of a gallbladder (GB) showing multiple internal echoes with a distinct echo (arrow) associated with an acoustic shadow (S). Only the echo with the accompanying shadow was considered to be a definite stone. This echo was produced by a single small calculus.

increased echogenicity of a calculus is to turn down the sensitivity setting. This reduces or even eliminates the echoes outlining the gallbladder wall and other soft-tissue structures. However, the stone echoes usually persist and are distinguished. Finally, gallbladder calculi are rounded or irregular in shape. The operator should be highly vigilant to contour changes produced by the gallstones. These changes may provide a scalloped appearance. Such irregularities usually make the inner echogenic zone of the calculi easy to discriminate from echoes of the gallbladder wall.

BILE DUCT EVALUATION

Operative diagnostic procedures for the common duct are designed to assist the surgeon in deciding when to perform a choledochotomy to explore the common and hepatic bile ducts. Without such diagnostic procedures, the surgeon could only rely on information from the history, physical examination, and preoperative diagnostic studies and on the gross findings at operation. The information from these sources may identify risk factors that suggest the likelihood of choledocholithiasis.

Risk factors vary in their capacity to predict with certainty the presence of common duct stones. One finding that is regarded with certainty is the presence of palpable stones in the common duct. This is viewed as an absolute indication for common duct exploration. Less certain risk factors have been considered as relative indications for common duct exploration. They may be findings discovered either preoperatively or during the operation.

Preoperative factors include a history of jaundice, cholangitis, or pancreatitis; physical or laboratory evidence of jaundice; and radiologic or ultrasonic evidence suggesting bile duct dilation or calculi. Factors that may be found during operation include the presence of small calculi in the gallbladder; an "empty" but inflamed gallbladder, which suggests passage of calculi; cystic duct dilation; and common duct dilation. Because choledochotomy and exploration are associated with a significantly increased morbidity and mortality, diagnostic procedures that may reduce the number of negative common duct explorations have been of interest to the biliary surgeon. The use of relative indications alone as the means for deciding which ducts to explore has resulted in a high negative exploration rate. Furthermore, stones in the common duct may be missed if none of the relative indications is evident. This problem led to the development and wide application of operative cholangiography as the principal means for assessing the common duct and for deciding which ducts to explore.[5]

Operative cholangiography is performed following the direct introduction of contrast material into the common duct either by using a fine gauge needle or, most commonly, by using a catheter passed through the cystic duct. A number of techniques entail fluoroscopy, film recording, or a combination of both procedures. Most surgeons employ the technique of contrast injection followed by exposure of two films.

Operative cholangiography has improved the surgeon's accuracy in deciding which common ducts to explore as compared with their accuracy when using risk factors alone in making this decision. However, cholangiography still misses some stone-bearing ducts and is associated with a false-positive rate of as high as 23%,[6] thereby leading to a high occurrence of negative explorations. This has raised questions about the cost-effectiveness of operative cholangiography.[6,7] For these reasons, operative ultrasonography may be used in conjunction with cholangiography in certain instances and as a possible replacement for operative cholangiography in other situations. A proposal for the use of operative ultrasound in conjunction with operative cholangiography or for its use without cholangiography as the initial screening test for the common duct is made later in this chapter.

Technique

Ultrasonography of the common bile duct should be performed after the duodenum has been mobilized by means of a Kocher maneuver and after the common hepatic and common bile ducts have been palpated.

The common bile duct, from the cystic duct junction to the superior margin of the duodenum, is examined first. Scanning is performed through

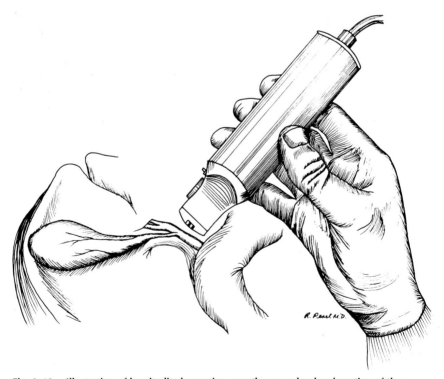

Fig. 4–10. Illustration of longitudinal scanning over the supraduodenal portion of the common bile duct.

the anterior aspect of the gastrohepatic ligament near its free edge (Fig. 4-10). The predominant scanning maneuvers are longitudinal scanning with transverse angulation. Maintenance of an acoustic window is essential to insure visualization of the entire duct.

The scanning of the common duct moves inferiorly over the anterior wall of the duodenum to image the distal or retroduodenal portion of the common duct. Transduodenal scanning of the retroduodenal portion of the common duct is the first of two maneuvers that are used to assess the terminal portion of the biliary duct (Fig. 4-11).

After completion of the transduodenal examination of the common bile duct, the duodenum should be retracted forward, and the retroduodenal portion of the common bile duct should be examined again from a postero-lateral approach (Fig. 4-12). The transducer-probe is pointed at the estimated location of the retroduodenal portion of the common duct. The transducer-probe may be placed across or along the long axis of the common duct. Placement is preferred along the long axis to longitudinally image the duct.

Because room for maneuvering the transducer-probe is usually limited, the two angulation maneuvers are primarily used to examine the retroduodenal portion of the common bile duct. Special attention must be given to

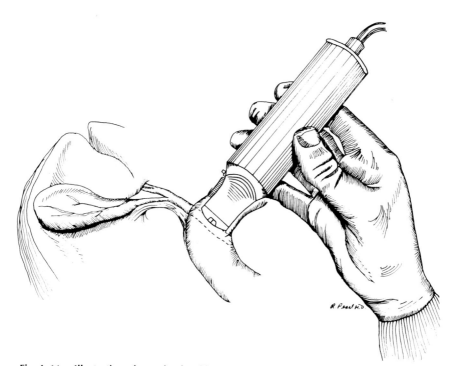

Fig. 4-11. Illustration of transduodenal longitudinal scanning demonstrates the retroduodenal portion of the common duct.

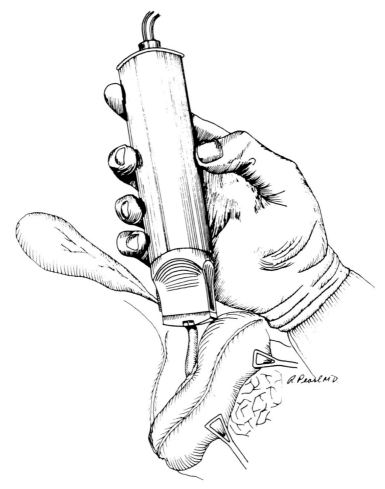

Fig. 4–12. Illustration of scanning maneuvers of the retroduodenal portion of the common bile duct using a posterior approach. The scanning is performed after the duodenum is mobilized and retracted anteromedially.

insuring that an acoustic window is maintained and that the lower portion of the duct is examined. This cannot be done unless the duodenum is mobilized and retracted anteromedially.

The common hepatic and the right and left hepatic ducts are examined last. The transducer-probe is placed longitudinally over the common hepatic duct just above the entrance of the cystic duct. Longitidunal scanning and transverse angulation are the predominant maneuvers as the transducer-probe is passed up to the confluence of the right and left hepatic ducts. At this point near the hilum of the liver, the transducer-probe is turned superiorly. The main hepatic radicals are scanned by using both the longitudinal and transverse angulation maneuvers (Fig. 4-13).

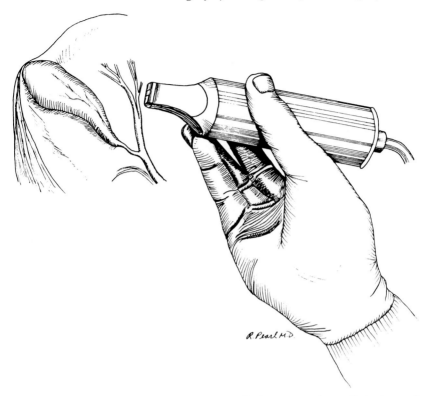

Fig. 4–13. Illustration of scanning of the hepatic radicals. Because of space limitations at the hepatic hilum, angulation maneuvers provide the best view. In the illustration, transverse angulation is being performed.

Findings

The normal common bile duct as imaged from the anterior aspect of the gastrohepatic ligament has a superficial location (Fig. 4-14). From this approach, the portal vein appears posterior to the duct. The caliber of the duct may be estimated from the sonographic image. The normal common duct is less than 1 cm wide near the entry of the cystic duct. As longitudinal scanning is performed distally through the duodenum, the terminal duct is seen to taper (Fig. 4-15).

Duct dilation can be detected by longitudinal scanning. Attention should be given to insuring that a small acoustic window is present and that the transducer-probe is positioned over the widest portion of the duct. If the ultrasound instrument has a range-measuring indicator, a precise estimate of caliber may be obtained. For more accurate estimation of size and a permanent record, a photograph of the monitor screen should be made for measurement.

Calculi within the common and hepatic ducts are recognized by using the same criteria as those used for recognizing gallbladder calculi. The operator

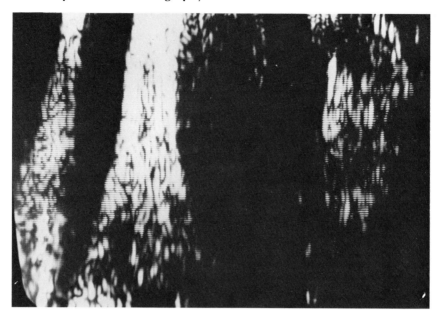

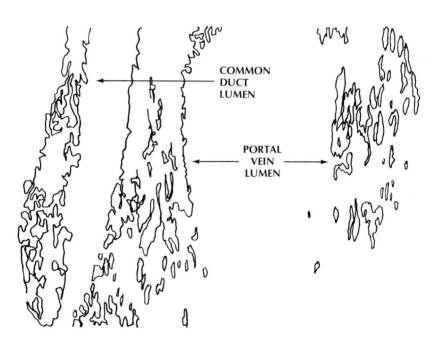

Fig. 4–14.   Sonogram of a longitudinal section through a normal common bile duct imaged through the anterior aspect of the gastrohepatic ligament. The portal vein is seen deep to the duct. (Reproduced from Sigel, B, et al.: Ultrasonic imaging during biliary and pancreatic surgery. Am J Surg, *141*:84, 1981.)

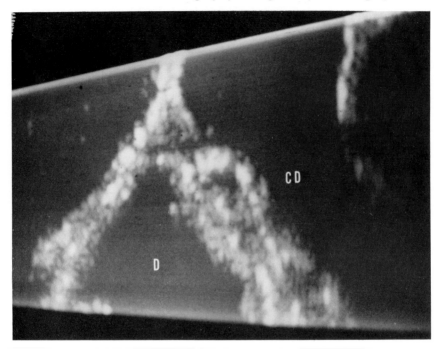

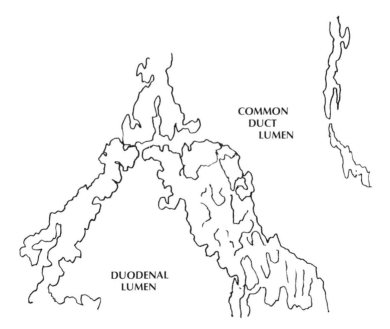

Fig. 4–15. Sonogram of a longitudinal section taken transduodenally to show the termination of the common bile duct (CD). The duct tapers in caliber in its inferior aspect. A portion of the duodenal lumen (D) is also seen.

should seek an echogenic outer zone and an acoustic shadow. The ultrasonic features of common duct stones vary according to their size, number, location, and echogenicity.

Small, highly echogenic stones are readily distinguished by the echogenic zone and acoustic shadow. When the common duct is dilated, care must be taken to demonstrate the acoustic shadow because it may be difficult to see in the sonolucent lumen of the duct (Fig. 4-16).

Calculi that are only moderately echogenic may be more difficult to detect than highly ecogenic stones. Not only are the surface echoes less distinct, but the acoustic shadow may also be less prominent. The operator should be aware of this possibility, particularly if ultrasonography of the gallbladder demonstrated moderately echogenic calculi (Fig. 4-17).

The detection of calculi in the distal common duct, particularly those that are impacted, requires special care because of the narrowness of the duct at this location. There is usually little or no duct lumen demonstrable between the superficial duct wall and the stone surface. Thus, a moderately echogenic stone may be difficult to distinguish from the ductal and duodenal walls. In these situations, an acoustic window must be maintained to make sure that the structures are not compressed. This window will facilitate the detection of an echogenic defect in the duct lumen. Another important sign of a calculus is the presence of an acoustic shadow—even one that is weak (Fig. 4-18).

In addition to detecting distinct calculi, ultrasonography may detect thickened bile (sludge), bile gravel, and cholesterol-fibrin casts.

Thickened bile may be detected in extrahepatic biliary obstruction due to noncalculus disease (e.g., malignancy). In this circumstance, the duct lumen shows a diffuse increase in echogenicity without discrete echogenicities or acoustic shadows indicating stones.

Bile gravel is the presence of multiple, small calculi in the bile that measure 1 or less millimeters in diameter. Unlike thickened bile, this type of bile produces a gritty sensation when rubbed over the finger tips. Gravel appears ultrasonically as multiple, small calculi. The dimension of the calculi is 1 millimeter or less, and they appear as ecogenic structures often with narrow acoustic shadows. Gallbladder debris consisting of fibrin and cholesterol may pass into the common bile duct. This material forms casts in the common duct and is less echogenic than calculi (Fig. 4-19).

Operative ultrasonography has been used during surgery for neonatal jaundice. A fusiform choleclochal cyst has been identified with this technique (Fig. 4-20).

The diagnosis of duct carcinoma can usually be made by inspection and palpation during operation. However, operative ultrasonography has been useful in demonstrating the extent of involvement. Extension of carcinoma into the common hepatic duct has been detected by ultrasonography (see Chap. 5, *Ultrasonography During Pancreatic Surgery*).

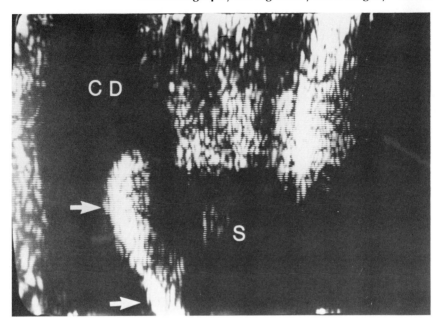

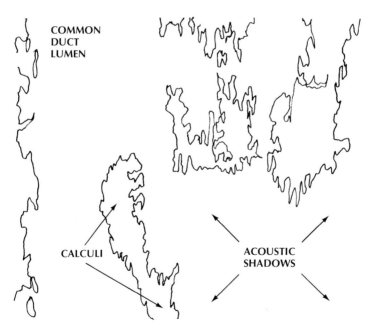

Fig. 4–16.   Sonogram of a longitudinal section through a dilated common bile duct (CD) shows two medium-sized echogenic calculi (arrows). Because the duct is dilated, the acoustic shadow (S) is difficult to distinguish in the duct lumen. It is best seen cutting across the posterior wall of the duct.

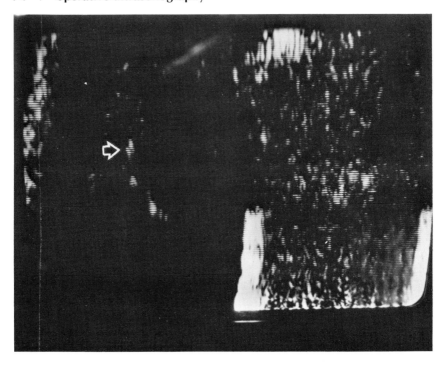

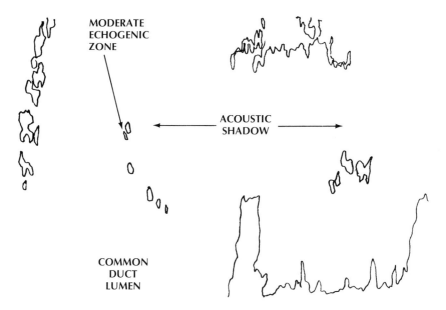

Fig. 4–17. Sonogram showing a longitudinal section of a dilated common bile duct. A moderately echogenic, large calculus is present (arrow). The acoustic shadow is less dense than that of a highly echogenic stone.

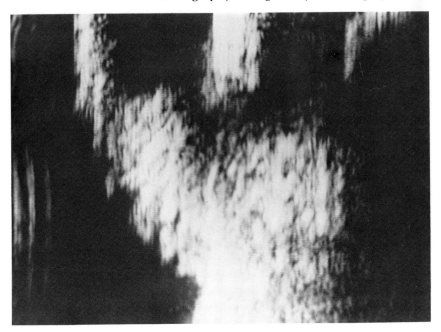

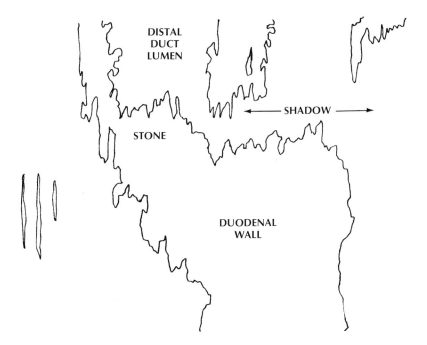

Fig. 4–18. Sonogram showing a longitudinal section of the distal common duct and duodenal wall. This stone is impacted, and its echoes are continuous with those of the duct wall and duodenum. The presence of a weak acoustic shadow helps to identify the stone.

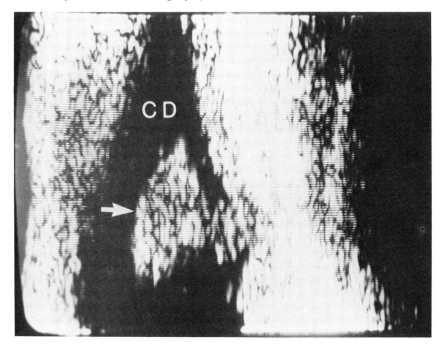

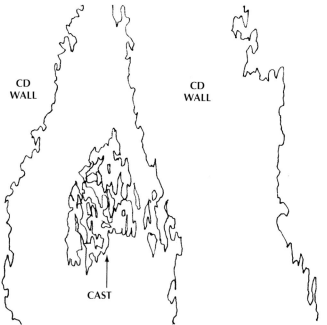

Fig. 4–19. Sonogram of a longitudinal section of a common duct (CD) containing a fibrin-cholesterol cast (arrow). The cast is irregular in shape and has approximately the same echogenicity as does the duct wall.

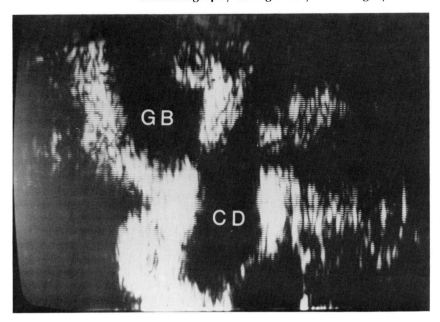

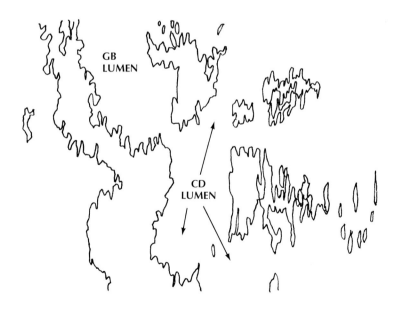

Fig. 4–20. Sonogram showing a gallbladder (GB) and a fusiform dilation of a common duct (CD) in an infant with neonatal jaundice.

RESULTS

Various findings and patterns of operative ultrasonography during biliary surgery have been described in the previous section. These have been qualitative assessments that have shown that operative ultrasound may help to locate the common duct when the anatomy has been distorted by previous inflammation or by operation, to detect the presence of gallbladder calculi, and to evaluate the common bile duct. A quantitative appraisal of ultrasound is more difficult to analyze for the first two applications than for the evaluation of the common bile duct. Our results are based on the first 129 patients to undergo ultrasonography of the biliary tract during operation.

In helping to locate a common duct in the midst of distorted anatomy, ultrasound is used in conjunction with operative exploration. When the ultrasound was used, the operator usually had sighted several locations as possibly containing the common duct. Ultrasonic scanning led to a surer and quicker selection of the correct site for the common bile duct.

In several situations, the opposite problem was encountered. The operator was so uncertain of the landmarks that the dissection proceeded slowly. Ultrasonic scanning helped to distinguish thickened peritoneum, fat, and connective tissue from bile duct and facilitated the search for the common duct.

During both types of situations—where the surgeon had identified several possible locations for the common duct and where a slow and tedious disection was underway—it was difficult to measure precisely the exact time saved or the amount of reduction of dissection provided by the ultrasound. However, the operating surgeon felt that ultrasonography did help to direct the search to locate the common duct and, on several occasions, indicated an unexpected close proximity to a previously unrecognized common duct.

Assessment of gallbladder content by operative palpation during exploration was also not always a clear-cut determination. In 18% of instances in which stones in the gallbladder were later confirmed by examining the removed gallbladder, palpation had failed to reveal the presence of stones. In another 20% of biliary operations, the gallbladder was ultimately proved to contain no calculi (these were instances of tumor obstruction of the bile ducts, stones having passed from the gallbladder, or acalculus cholecystitis). Operative ultrasound correctly diagnosed all instances in which stones were present but not palpable and all instances in which stones were not present in the gallbladder.

Another important result of gallbladder ultrasonography was the ability to confirm stone size. In a number of instances, calculi larger than 5 millimeters in diameter were diagnosed on preoperative studies or discovered by the operator on palpating the gallbladder. However, the presence of calculi measuring 2 to 3 millimeters in diameter frequently was not detected in the gallbladders. By indicating the presence of small stones early during the operation, ultrasound provided the surgeon with information that could be useful in determining whether to explore the common bile duct.

In our first 47 operations, we assessed the accuracy of operative ultrasonography compared with the accuracy of preoperative ultrasonography for gallbladder calculi.[8] There were no false-negative or false-positive results for the operative examination. Preoperative ultrasonography was associated with one false-negative and four false-positive examinations. Thus, operative ultrasonography was distinctly a more accurate examination than preoperative imaging.

More quantifiable results were obtained with the use of operative ultrasonography in the evaluation of the common bile duct. The ability to obtain such information is particularly pertinent because the most important application of operative ultrasonography in biliary surgery is the evaluation of the common duct for presence of stones. As previously mentioned, the results to be presented are based on our first 129 patients to undergo operative ultrasonography of the common duct. These patients represent a selection that was biased to produce a higher prevalence of common duct calculi. Often, we were unable to perform ultrasonography in all biliary operations performed on the same day. When given a choice between performing operative ultrasonography in a patient with preoperative risk factors for common duct calculi and in a patient without risk factors, we usually selected the patient with the greater likelihood of a common duct disorder. In evauating results, a comparison was made between ultrasonography and cholangiography in helping to formulate the decision to explore the common bile duct. The results are summarized in Table 4-1.

TABLE 4-1

Comparison of Operative Ultrasound and Operative Cholangiography in Detecting Common Duct Calculi

	Ultrasonography	Cholangiography
True-Negative	99	77
True-Positive	23	19
False-Negative	3	2
False-Positive	4	7
Not Performed	—	22
Technically Unsatisfactory	—	2
	129	129
Sensitivity	$\dfrac{23}{23 + 3} = 89\%$	$\dfrac{19}{19 + 2} = 91\%$
Specificity	$\dfrac{99}{99 + 4} = 96\%$	$\dfrac{77}{77 + 7} = 92\%$
Efficiency	$\dfrac{23 + 99}{23 + 99 + 3 + 4} = 95\%$	$\dfrac{19 + 77}{19 + 77 + 2 + 7} = 91\%$
Predictive value of a positive test	$\dfrac{23}{23 + 4} = 85\%$	$\dfrac{19}{19 + 7} = 73\%$
Predictive value of a negative test	$\dfrac{99}{99 + 3} = 97\%$	$\dfrac{77}{77 + 2} = 97\%$

Table 4-1 shows the results on the basis of true negative, true positive, false-negative, and false-positive findings. In the three false-negative ultrasonic examinations, the cholangiograms were positive, and subsequent duct exploration confirmed the presence of stones. One of these errors occurred early in our experience. Another appeared to be the result of inadequate mobilization of the duodenum, which prevented a complete ultrasonic examination of the retroduodenal common duct. In one false-positive ultrasound examination, calculi were mistakenly believed to be present in the common duct when, in reality, they were in a dilated cystic duct that was parallel to and intimately adherent to the common duct. During three other operations, small echoes believed to represent gravel were found in the common duct. Following choledochotomy, no calculi were found.

In one false-negative cholangiogram, ultrasonography revealed a 3-by-8 millimeter cast composed of cholesterol and fibrin. This was observed on ultrasonography, and on this basis, the duct was opened and the cast removed. In another instance, a small stone was missed by cholangiography but detected by ultrasound.

In seven patients, the cholangiogram was falsely positive. In four of these instances, the operative ultrasonograms revealed no calculi. In one instance, a small filling defect was observed on cholangiography. Real-time ultrasonography showed that the defect was produced by a small pulsating indention that was probably the right hepatic artery. The duct was not explored, a postoperative intravenous cholangiogram was normal, and the patient's course was uneventful. In a second patient, dye failed to enter the duodenum on both cholangiographic films. Because of the normal ultrasonogram, the cholangiography was repeated following glucagon administration producing a normal study and sparing the patient a negative duct exploration. In a third patient, cholangiography revealed the same filling defects following two injections of the contrast material. In view of the normal ultrasound examination, yet another contrast injection was made. This time, the duct was entirely normal suggesting a bubble artifact on the previous films. Duct exploration was avoided. In a fourth false-positive cholangiogram, a filling defect was seen but ultrasonography was negative. The duct was opened, but the exploration was negative. The results in Table 4-1 are analyzed in terms of sensitivity, specificity, efficiency, predictive value of a positive test and predictive value of a negative test. These are indices for measuring the validity of diagnostic tests and are defined (together with prevalence) as follows:

$$\text{Sensitivity} = \frac{\text{True-Positives (TP)} \times 100}{\text{True-Positives (TP)} + \text{False-Negatives (FN)}}$$

$$\text{Specificity} = \frac{\text{True-Negatives (TN)} \times 100}{\text{True-Negatives (TN)} + \text{False-Positives (FP)}}$$

$$\text{Efficiency} = \frac{[\text{True-Positives (TP)} + \text{True-Negatives (TN)}] \times 100}{\text{TP} + \text{TN} + \text{FP} + \text{FN}}$$

$$\begin{matrix}\text{Predictive Value of} \\ \text{a Positive Test}\end{matrix} = \frac{\text{True-Positives (TP)} \times 100}{\text{True-Positives (TP)} + \text{False-Positives (FP)}}$$

$$\begin{matrix}\text{Predictive Value of} \\ \text{a Negative Test}\end{matrix} = \frac{\text{True-Negatives (TN)} \times 100}{\text{True-Negatives (TN)} + \text{False-Negatives (FN)}}$$

$$\text{Prevalence} = \frac{[\text{True-Positives (TP)} + \text{False-Negatives (FN)}] \times 100}{\text{TP} + \text{TN} + \text{FP} + \text{FN}}$$

Sensitivity, specificity, and efficiency measure the accuracy of a diagnostic test without taking into account how often the abnormality for which the test is performed occurs in the population being examined. Sensitivity of a test is a trait intended to identify any reasonable possibility of abnormality. Since the definition of "reasonable" may vary, the level of the sensitivity must be arbitrarily set to screen a large population. The purpose is to identify a smaller sample with greater likelihood of having the abnormality. Specificity of a test is the certainty with which a negative test may be used to exclude the presence of the abnormality. Efficiency is the combined measure of test accuracy based on both sensitivity and specificity.

The predictive value of a positive test indicates to the user how often the abnormality is really present when the test is positive. This test is dependent on the prevalence or occurrence of the abnormality in the total population being examined. The reason for the test's prevalence-dependent characteristic can be seen from examining the definition. The denominator of the predictive value of a positive test fraction contains both true-positive and false-positive occurrences. If the false-positive rate is high (low specificity) and if there are many instances of no abnormality in the population (low prevalence), the *total* number of false-positives will be large. This tends to lower the predictability of a positive test.

The prevalence of common duct calculi is relatively low. The 20.0% figure in our experience is hgher than that in most reported series because of preference given to inclusion of patients with risk factors. Yet, this prevalence produces a predictive value of a positive test based on risk factors of about 52%. The predictive values of a positive test for operative ultrasonography and for operative cholangiography are 85% and 73%, respectively. These figures would be lesser if the prevalence were lower.

In our series of patients, there was one instance of retained stones following exploration. Both ultrasonography and cholangiography were positive. Several stones in the hepatic radicals could not be removed during operation or during postoperative choledochal endoscopy. These stones were removed during a second operation. There was no operative mortality in this group of patients.

CONCLUSIONS

Operative ultrasonography during biliary surgery has three main uses. Ultrasonography may be helpful in locating the common bile duct where anatomy has been distorted by previous inflammation or operation. Assessment of gallbladder content for the presence of calculi may be made with 100% accuracy. This may aid in the detection of calculi in gallbladders that are distended, have thickened walls, or are surrounded by adhesions precluding adequate palpation. Furthermore, small stones that may not have been detected by preoperative testing or operative palpation may be discovered by operative ultrasonography. This information could be important in a decision regarding possible exploration of the common bile duct.

The principal application of operative ultrasonography is the evaluation of the common bile duct. Favorable results with the use of operative ultrasound in biliary surgery have been reported.[1,8,9,10] The sensitivity, specificity, and predictive value of a negative test of operative ultrasound and operative cholangiography are comparable. False-positives and false-negatives occur with either test.

Thus, neither test gives perfect results. The predictive value of a positive test for operative cholangiography is lower than for operative ultrasonography. This tends to cause a relatively higher negative common duct exploration rate. Since the tests are somewhat complementary, decision strategies should be devised that combine the information provided to enhance the positive rate of common duct exploration without increasing the rate of missed stones.

Only one false-negative and no false-positives occurred in patients with low risk for choledocholithiasis (no jaundice or duct dilation) who were examined by ultrasonography. The one false-negative consisted of a single 3-mm stone. Cholangiography produced one false-negative and four false-positive results in this category of patients. Thus, it may be reasonable to conclude that, for the patients at low risk for common duct stones, operative ultrasonography may appropriately be used as the sole screening operative diagnostic procedure. The substitution of operative ultrasonography for operative cholangiography in lower-risk patients provides the advantage of less dissection and operating time and the avoidance of contrast material and radiation exposure.

RECOMMENDED APPLICATIONS

1. Operative ultrasonography may be usefully employed to locate more quickly and safely the common bile duct when right upper quadrant anatomy has been distorted by previous inflammation or operation.

2. Operative ultrasonography may be used to detect the presence of gallbladder calculi when such information cannot be obtained by palpation

because of a distended gallbladder, a gallbladder with thickened walls, or a gallbladder surrounded by adhesions. In operations for known biliary calculi, this technique can provide information about the number, location, and size of the calculi. In operations for nonbiliary conditions in which preoperative tests for calculi were not performed, ultrasonography may establish the diagnosis. In either instance, operative ultrasonography of the gallbladder may confirm the presence and size of calculi and may provide information for decisions regarding the need for cholecystectomy and common duct exploration.

3. Operative ultrasonography should be used in conjunction with operative cholangiography in making a decision about common duct exploration in patients at increased risk for common duct stones. Increased risk is defined as the presence of one or more preoperative or operative risk factors for choledocholithiasis. The risk factors include jaundice, pancreatitis, small calculi in the gallbladder or cystic duct, dilated cystic duct, and dilated common duct. The following actions are recommended for each of four possible contingencies:

A. Ultrasound and cholangiography both negative. The common duct should not be explored.

B. Ultrasound and cholangiography both positive. The common duct should be explored.

C. Ultrasound is positive, but cholangiography is negative. The common duct should be explored.

D. Ultrasound is negative, but cholangiography is positive. If a compressive defect is present, careful observation of real-time imaging should be performed to rule out compression by a pulsating artery. If the contrast material fails to enter the duodenum on the initial study, the repeat injection of contrast material should be made after the administration of glucagon. If the abnormality cannot be explained or does not clear on repeat cholangiography, the common duct should be explored.

4. Operative ultrasonography may be used as a substitute for operative cholangiography in patients who do not show any risk factors suggesting choledochlithiasis. If ultrasonography is negative, the common duct need not be explored. If ultrasonography is positive, cholangiography and common duct exploration should be performed. In these low-risk common ducts, operative ultrasonography may serve as the screening test for choledocholithiasis.

5
ULTRASONOGRAPHY DURING PANCREATIC SURGERY

Ultrasound scanning may be employed during operations on the pancreas for both malignancy and inflammatory disease.[9,10] A variety of applications have been made that either further define the diagnostic information of preoperative testing or provide new information that was not obtained or was not obtainable prior to surgery. For suspected pancreatic or periampullary neoplasms, operative ultrasonography may be used to evaluate the location and extent of the tumor and the status of the biliary and pancreatic ducts. For inflammatory disease, sonography may be used in surgery for pancreatic abscess, pseudocyst, and chronic pancreatitis.

This chapter considers each of the uses in terms of techniques, findings, and overall results. Based on this experience, conclusions are drawn and specific applications are recommended for the surgeon operating on the pancreas.

TECHNIQUE AND ULTRASONIC APPEARANCE OF NORMAL PANCREAS

The pancreas may be examined during the operation by ultrasound scanning through the gastrocolic ligament or, more directly, after the gastrocolic ligament has been transected. The technique to be used whenever possible and the findings of the examination of a normal gland are described in this section. Afterward, ultrasonography during operation for pancreatic tumors and inflammatory disease will be considered.

Technique

The initial maneuver in the ultrasonic examination of the pancreas should be several longitudinal scans with transverse angulation. The paths for each longitudinal scan should be roughly parallel and about 1 centimeter apart. Longitudinal scanning along the superior half of the pancreas should identify the splenic artery and vein. Following this maneuver, the head should be re-examined using transverse scanning. This step identifies the distal-most portion of the common duct near the duodenum. As the transducer-probe is moved to the patient's left side, the superior mesenteric vein and artery should be seen (Fig. 5-1).

During pancreatic scanning, an acoustic window of ½ to 1 centimeter must be maintained. This permits recognition of surface irregularities, maintains better orientation, and prevents compression of ducts and blood vessels.

Findings

Figure 5-2 is a sonogram showing a section of pancreas obtained by longitudinal scanning along the body of a normal gland. The anterior

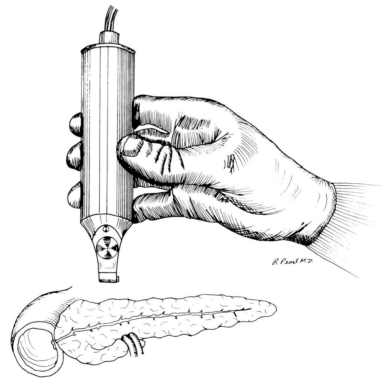

Fig. 5–1. Illustration showing transverse scanning of the pancreas in the region of the superior mesenteric vessels.

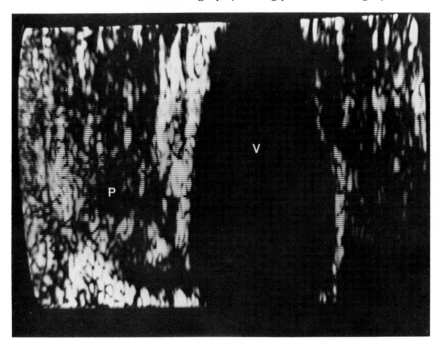

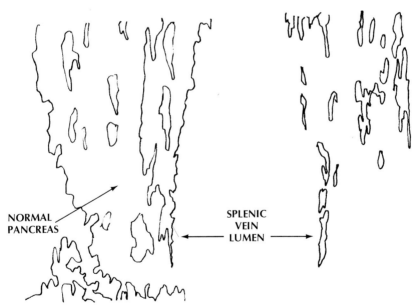

NORMAL
PANCREAS

SPLENIC
VEIN
LUMEN

Fig. 5–2. Sonogram of a longitudinal section through a normal pancreas. Pancreatic tissue (P) demonstrates the fine recticular pattern of the small pancreatic ducts. The splenic vein (V) is seen deep to the pancreatic tissue. (Reproduced from Sigel, B: Ultrasonic imaging during biliary and pancreatic surgery. Am J Surg, *141*:84, 1981.)

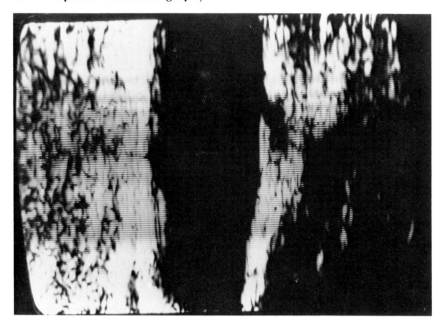

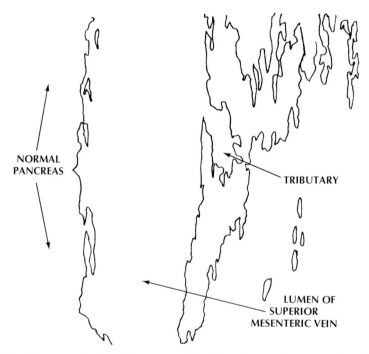

Fig. 5–3. Sonogram showing a transverse section through a normal pancreas. Deep to the pancreatic tissue is the superior mesenteric vein, which is receiving a tributary on its deep surface

surface, gland substance, and splenic vein can be discerned. The normal gland shows moderately echogenic parenchyma interspersed with an intertwining network of fine sonolucent structures representing the reticulum of small pancreatic ducts. The main pancreatic ducts are 2 to 4 millimeters in diameter.

Figure 5-3 is a sonogram of a transverse scan at the junction of the head and body of the pancreas. The superior mesenteric vein with a small tributary that enters posteriorly is seen deep to the gland substance.

SURGERY FOR PANCREATIC AND PERIAMPULLARY TUMORS

During an operation for suspected pancreatic malignant tumor, a number of management decisions are usually necessary. These decisions require information that is related directly to the tumor and to the secondary effects of the tumor on the biliary and pancreatic ducts.

Initially, the diagnosis must be confirmed. In the absence of metastases or extension of the tumor outside the pancreas, an enlargement in the pancreas must be determined to be a malignant tumor or chronic pancreatitis. This may be a problem because the two entities may produce tissue enlargement and induration, and tumor is frequently associated with chronic pancreatitis. Operative ultrasonography cannot distinguish between tumor and pancreatitis. However, ultrasound can provide information that, when considered with other findings, may assist in making a decision for or against extirpative surgery.

Technique

In patients with jaundice and dilation of the biliary ducts, operative ultrasonography should be used to examine completely the gallbladder and biliary ducts in a manner similar to that described in the previous chapter (see Chap. 4, *Ultrasonography During Biliary Tract Surgery*).

The pancreas should be exposed through the gastrocolic ligament. Following inspection and palpation, ultrasound examination should be performed as described previously in this chapter. In an area of suspected tumor, additional longitudinal and transverse scanning maneuvers should be done (Fig. 5-4).

Biopsy of the pancreas is a controversial issue. Some surgeons believe that an attempt to establish a tissue diagnosis should be made prior to performing an extensive surgical procedure, such as removal of the duodenum and pancreas. Other surgeons believe that attempts to establish a tissue diagnosis at operation are too inaccurate and pose sufficient additional risk to the patient to justify an attempt to remove the tumor without a tissue diagnosis.

Should a decision for needle biopsy of a suspected pancreatic neoplasm be made, operative ultrasonography may be used to guide the needle. Needle biopsy may be made directly into pancreatic tissue (Fig. 5-5). An alternative technique, which we prefer, is to pass the needle first through the

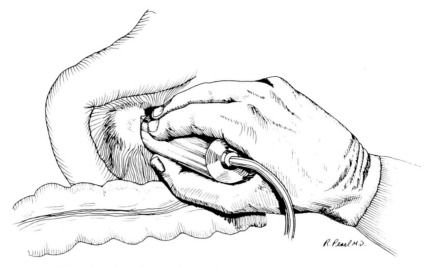

Fig. 5–4. Illustration of an ultrasound scan of a tumor in the head of the pancreas.

duodenum and then into the pancreas. The intent with either approach is to avoid puncture of a blood vessel or a dilated pancreatic duct. Prior to biopsy, the pancreas, at a prospective site, is scanned to determine the location of solid echogenic tissue. Such surveillance determines the exact point of placement of the biopsy needle and the anticipated direction of the needle path through pancreatic tissue. Scanning is continued while the needle is passed to keep large blood vessels and dilated pancreatic ducts in view.

Detection of tumor invasion of the superior mesenteric and portal veins is achieved by scanning these structures through the substance of the pancreas. An acoustic window must be maintained, and the surface of the gland must not be contacted. Even slight pressure from the transducer may compress the veins and prevent detection of venous narrowing or invasion.

Findings

Examination of the biliary system in patients with jaundice associated with a pancreatic or periampullary mass may provide positive and negative information, both of which may help in the overall assessment of the condition. Positive information includes the confirmation of duct dilation with a precise estimate of the degree of dilation. In addition, ultrasound may reveal an image pattern suggestive of ductal obstruction produced by tumors. A negative finding, which is useful in excluding other disease, is the absence of biliary calculi in the gallbladder and biliary ducts.

Operative ultrasonography may reveal bile duct dilation that may not have been fully appreciated by inspection alone. The caliber of the duct may be obtained by estimating dimensions on the monitor or by using a range-measuring indicator (if present on the ultrasound instrument).

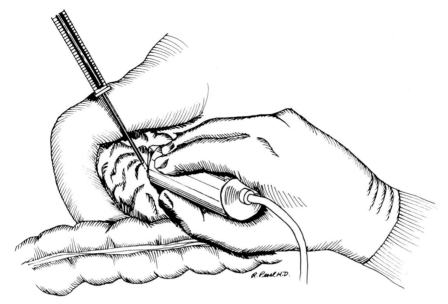

Fig. 5–5.   Illustration showing technique for ultrasonic guidance of a biopsy needle into the pancreas.

The image pattern of common duct termination in obstruction may be discerned by ultrasonography and may provide inferential evidence of tumor as the cause of the obstruction. We have observed two types of common duct terminations produced by tumor. One pattern is a tapered narrowing of the common bile duct occurring at a site proximal to the normal duct tapering produced by the sphincter of Oddi (Fig. 5-6). This narrowing is characteristic of extrinsic compression of the duct produced by a carcinoma of the pancreatic head. Another pattern is a tumor-shelf deformity or ledge produced by intraductal infiltration of tumor (Figs. 5-7 and 5-8).

The absence of biliary calculi within a large distended gallbladder and dilated common bile duct helps to rule out calculus disease. Although this absence does not establish a diagnosis of biliary obstruction produced by tumor, the lack of stones is a factor favoring such a diagnosis. At times, biliary calculi may be present in association with a pancreatic or periampullary malignancy. Such calculi may not be detected by palpation because of the distention of the gallbladder and bile ducts. In such circumstances, operative ultrasonography or cholangiography may be required to demonstrate these calculi.

The ultrasonic appearance of pancreatic tumors may show tissue with increased echogenicity. However, the most consistent finding that we noted was an absence of the network of fine sonolucent ducts and their replacement by duct dilation. Ducts measuring ½ to 1 centimeter in caliber were frequently seen (Fig. 5-9).

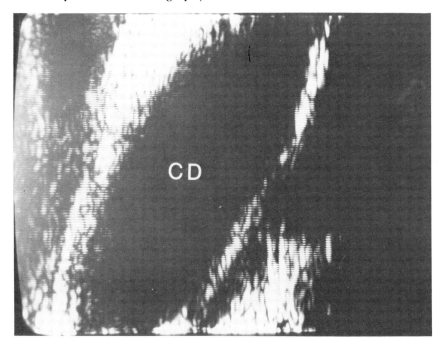

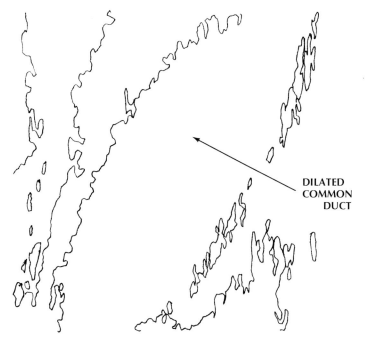

Fig. 5–6. Sonogram showing a longitudinal section through a dilated common duct (CD) containing no calculi.

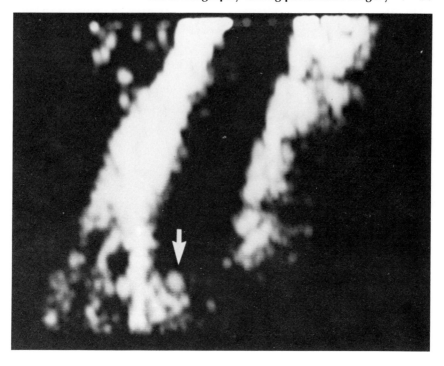

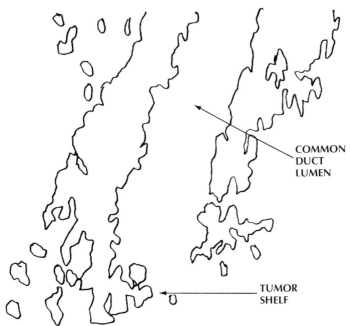

COMMON
DUCT
LUMEN

TUMOR
SHELF

Fig. 5–7. Sonogram showing a longitudinal section through a common duct with an infiltrating tumor that produces an obstructing shelf (arrow).

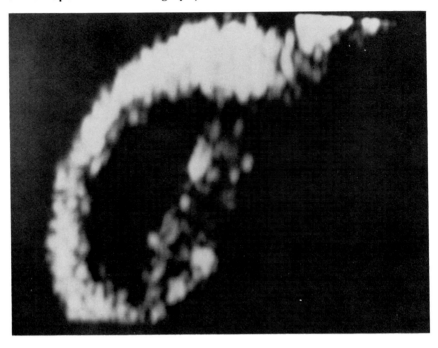

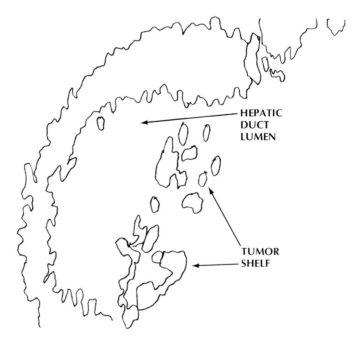

Fig. 5–8. Sonogram showing a transverse section through a dilated common hepatic duct. A tumor shelf can be seen to occupy about one-half the lumen of the duct.

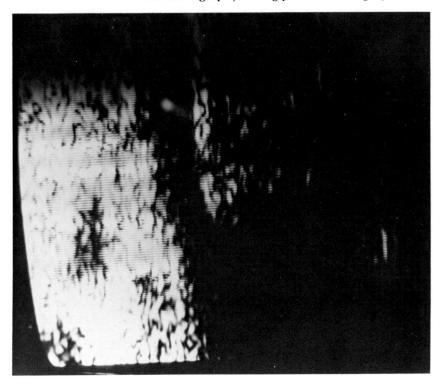

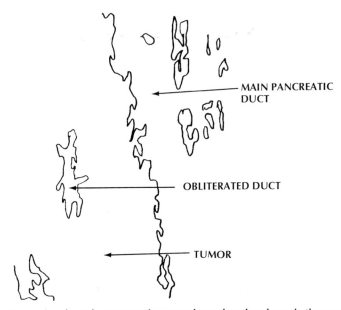

MAIN PANCREATIC DUCT

OBLITERATED DUCT

TUMOR

Fig. 5–9. Sonogram through a pancreatic tumor shows densely echogenic tissue encasing and obliterating some ducts. The main pancreatic duct is deep to the tumor and appears to be dilated slightly.

The close proximity of dilated pancreatic ducts to areas of suspected tumor illustrates the problem of pancreatic tumor biopsy. When a decision was made to perform a biopsy of a suspected tumor, ultrasonic guidance of a biopsy needle helped to avoid inadvertent puncture of blood vessels and dilated ducts.

Tumor involvement of the superior mesenteric and portal veins may be recognized by the presence of several signs. Normal veins, when imaged by

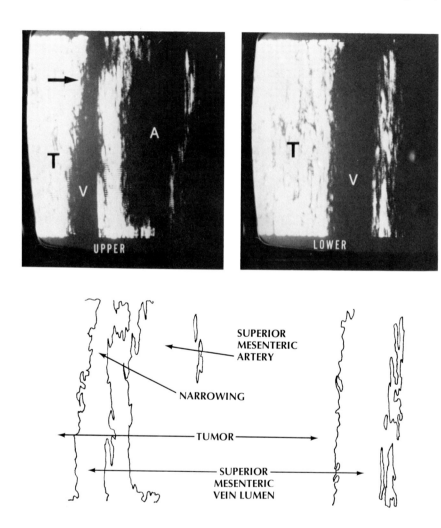

Fig. 5–10. Composite of two sonograms showing pancreatic tumor (T) and the superior mesenteric vein (V). The sonogram on the left is of a higher segment of the vein and shows a narrowing of the vein by tumor (T). The narrowing is most marked at the arrow. The superior mesenteric artery (A) is also seen with tissue of increased echogenicity encroaching on both vessels. The sonogram on the right shows a lower segment of the vein; the tumor (T) is not compressing the vein (V).

real-time scanning, are seen to change caliber with the patient's respiration. Failure to observe this fluctuation in size is suggestive of perivenous infiltration. Other signs of tumor involvement are narrowing of a venous segment and intraluminal extension by the tumor (Fig. 5-10). If none of these signs is present, the surgeon has reasonable assurance that the superior mesenteric-portal vein axis is free of tumor involvement. In addition, ultrasonography can precisely locate the veins when their presence is not readily detected. This ability should help the surgeon during the dissection of these veins away from the pancreas.

SURGERY FOR INFLAMMATORY DISEASE OF THE PANCREAS

Although surgery on the pancreas may not be needed in acute and relatively mild episodes of pancreatitis, surgery is often required for the complications of pancreatitis, such as abscess, pseudocyst, and chronic pancreatitis. Recent developments in ultrasonography, endoscopic cholangiopancreatography, and computerized tomography have aided in the management of these complications by making it possible, in most instances, to establish a diagnosis preoperatively. Ultrasonography has been employed during operations for these complications of pancreatitis to confirm the diagnosis and to facilitate the performance of certain operative maneuvers.

In pancreatic abscess, operative ultrasound may be used to confirm abscess cavities and to locate precisely these cavities in terms of landmarks visible to the surgeon. Confirmation works in two ways: it identifies an abscess cavity when it is there and it rules out a cavity in instances of pancreatic enlargement or surrounding tissue swelling produced by inflammatory edema. Patients with such disorders are usually febrile and very ill. For this reason, diagnostic assistance that expedites the establishment of external drainage and shortens operating time may be of considerable importance.

In pancreatic pseudocyst, operative ultrasound may be used to confirm the presence of a cystic cavity just as it may be used to identify an abscess cavity. In pseudocyst surgery, however, the usual objective of the operation is to establish adequate internal drainage instead of external drainage. This requires not only an appraisal of the size and extent of the pseudocyst but often a selection of the ideal site for drainage of the cyst into the gastrointestinal tract. Selection of a drainage site is determined by the location that would insure adequate drainage and avoid injury to adjacent structures. In addition, information regarding cyst-wall thickness may aid in the selection of the optimal wall thickness for suture placement. As with pancreatic abscess, confirmation of the presence of a pseudocyst also works in two ways: it detects cysts when they are present and rules out their presence when an area of enlargement is caused by inflammatory swelling. In this way, needless needle aspiration or exploration may be avoided.

In chronic pancreatitis, operative ultrasound may be used to determine the condition and location of the pancreatic ducts. Once a decision has been made to operate on a patient with chronic pancreatitis, the status of pancreatic ducts is an important factor in confirming the diagnosis and selecting the appropriate operation. There is controversy regarding the type of operation to perform for chronic pancreatitis. If the pancreatic ductal system is significantly dilated secondary to obstruction, an internal drainage procedure into the intestinal tract may be performed. Another approach is to remove a part or most of the gland. Our preference is to attempt to do an internal drainage operation as described by Puestow, particularly if dilation of the ductal system is significant. We would consider partial or subtotal resection if pancreatic ducts could not be found or if a previous internal drainage operation had not succeeded. Operative ultrasonography has been of assistance during surgery for chronic pancreatitis by confirming and specifically localizing the site of dilated ducts. Conversely, ultrasound may be used to exclude the presence of duct dilation. In this way, it may help with the decision to perform a pancreatic resection instead of an internal drainage operation.

Technique

In patients with suspected pancreatic abscess, any masses or enlargements should be examined by ultrasound. Abscesses may be multiple or may extend to considerable distances from the pancreas. All abscess cavities and all extensions must be located and drained completely.

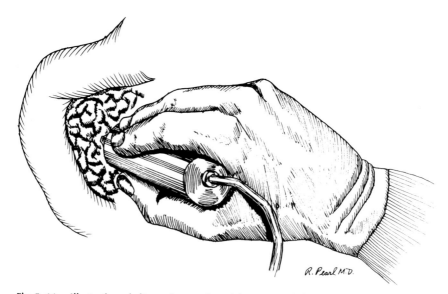

Fig. 5–11. Illustration of ultrasonic scanning of the pancreatic head through the gastrocolic ligament.

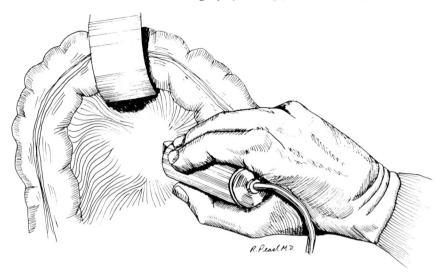

R. Pearl M.D.

Fig. 5–12. Illustration of ultrasonic scanning of a pseudocyst through the transverse mesocolon.

Ultrasonography for abscess should be performed at the time of the initial exploration. The usual ultrasonic scanning directly on the gland may not be possible because the gastrocolic ligament is adherent to the gland as a result of inflammation and adhesion formation. Any bulging and accessible peritoneal surface should be scanned. This could be the gastrohepatic or gastrocolic ligaments, the transverse mesocolon, or the base of the small bowel mesentery or posterior peritoneum. After an abscess is found and drained, any remaining swellings should be re-examined by ultrasound to insure that drainage is complete.

During operations for pancreatic pseudocyst, any mass discovered at initial exploration should be ultrasonically scanned through the most accessible peritoneal surface. This approach is similar to that used for pancreatic abscess and may entail imaging through the gastrocolic ligament (Fig. 5-11) or through the transverse mesocolon (Fig. 5-12). A search should be made for extrapancreatic extension of the pseudocyst.

If the lesser peritoneal space is not obliterated, the pancreas should be exposed by transecting the gastrocolic ligament. The surface of the gland can then be inspected, palpated, and ultrasonically scanned. This may be done rapidly by longitudinal scanning maneuvers. If a mass is located in the pancreatic head, scanning may be performed from the lateral aspect of the pancreatic head posterior to the duodenum, which may be displaced anteriorly (Fig. 5-13).

If the pseudocyst is behind the stomach and cystgastrostomy is being considered, the pseudocyst may be scanned through the back wall of the stomach after an opening is made in the anterior gastric wall.

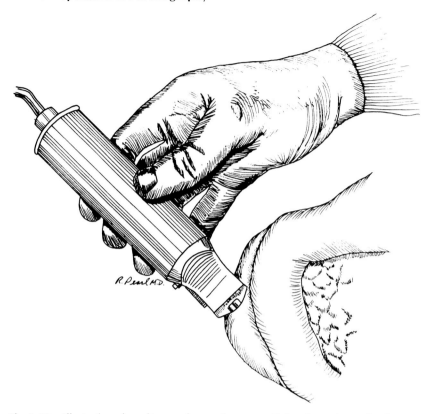

R. Pearl M.D.

Fig. 5–13. Illustration of an ultrasound scan of a pancreatic head pseudocyst that has displaced the duodenum anteriorly. The approach is from the lateral aspect of the mass.

During operations for chronic pancreatitis, ultrasonic examination is best performed after the gland is exposed by transection of the gastrocolic ligament. Both longitudinal and transverse scanning maneuvers may be used to locate dilated ducts (Fig. 5-14). Once dilated ducts have been confirmed and a decision for an internal drainage operation has been made, ultrasound guidance of an aspirating needle may be performed to locate and enter more precisely the main pancreatic duct.

Findings

In patients with suspected abscess, operative ultrasonography has been used to discern the contents of masses and to help to identify extension of abscess cavities. Areas of inflammation and necrosis may be recognized by their diffuse echogenic patterns, which is distinct from areas of relative sonolucency characteristic of abscess cavities. The boundary between an abscess wall and the abscess cavity is usually not sharp. The wall may be irregular or, more frequently, there may be a graded transition from the

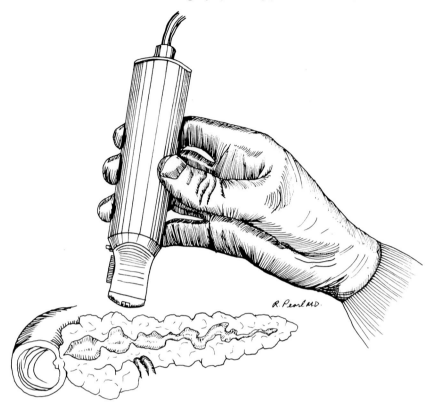

Fig. 5–14. Illustration of longitudinal scanning of the surface of the pancreas to locate dilated ducts associated with chronic pancreatitis.

echogenic area representing the wall to the more sonolucent abscess cavity. Figure 5-15 shows the indistinct transition from the abscess wall to the cavity in a section made through the transverse mesocolon. Multiple small cavities were seen in close proximity to the main abscess cavity. One of these cavities can be seen in the sonogram and is situated within the thickened mesocolon. The smaller satellite cavities were found to communicate with the main abscess cavity.

In patients with pancreatic pseudocyst, the ultrasonic distinction between wall and cavity is usually more clearly defined than that in abscess. In addition, the cystic cavity, because of less debris, is more sonolucent than an abscess cavity (Figs. 5-16 and 5-17). A number of important observations may be made with operative ultrasound during surgery for pseudocyst. These include confirmation of the diagnosis, location of adjacent structures, and determination of cyst-wall thickness.

Confirmation of a pseudocyst is achieved by demonstrating a fluid locula-tion in the pancreas or in an adjacent or nearby enlargement. Operative ultrasonography can distinguish cystic areas from masses produced by in-

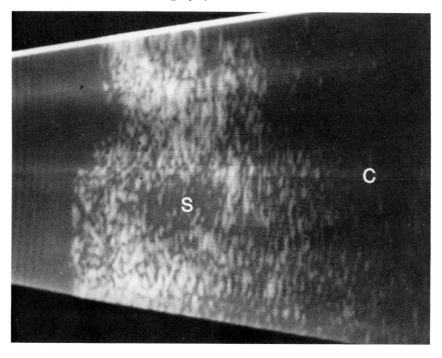

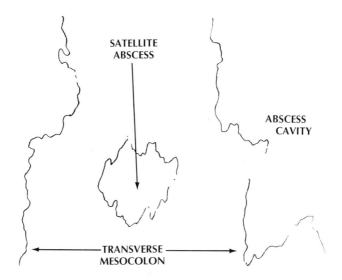

Fig. 5–15. Sonogram of a pancreatic abscess taken through the transverse mesocolon. The distinction between the abscess wall and cavity (C) is not clear. A small satellite abscess (S) is located within the thickened mesocolon.

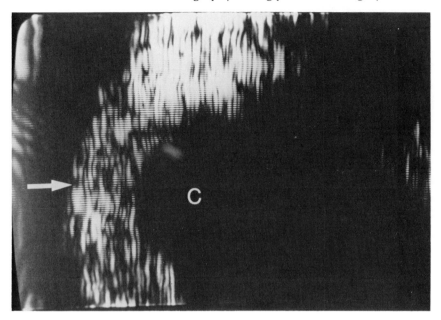

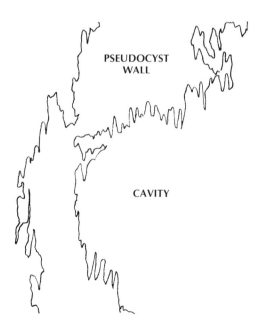

Fig. 5–16. Sonogram showing a pancreatic pseudocyst. The wall of the cyst (arrow) is sharply delineated from the cystic cavity (C).

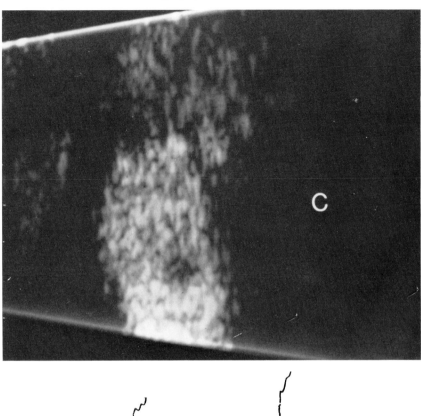

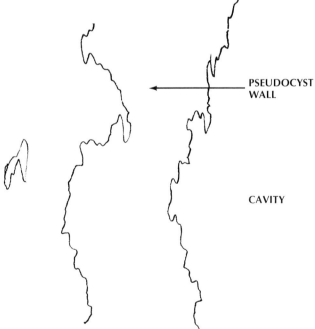

PSEUDOCYST
WALL

CAVITY

Fig. 5–17. Sonogram of a pancreatic pseudocyst in the tail of the pancreas. C is the cavity of the pseudocyst.

flammatory edema. Figure 5-18 shows sonograms of sections through two areas of enlargement of the pancreas found at the same operation. One area with internal echoes throughout was interpreted to represent inflammatory edema, whereas the other area was considered to show a pseudocyst. Needle aspiration proved both interpretations to be correct.

The structures most commonly identified by ultrasonography in previously unrecognized close proximity to pancreatic pseudocysts are the duodenum and major blood vessels. Figure 5-19 shows a fluid-filled duodenum in close contact to a pseudocyst of the pancreatic head. The cyst had expanded posteriorly and laterally to the duodenum. The location of the duodenum was revealed by the ultrasound scan. Further inspection and dissection verified the anterior and medial displacement of the duodenal sweep. The location of the duodenum was obscured by a combination of displacement plus compression by the pseudocyst, and the defacement of normal landmarks was caused by inflammation.

Figure 5-20 is a sonogram showing the splenic artery in proximity to the lumen of a pseudocyst posterior to the stomach. After the stomach was opened, the cyst was scanned through the posterior gastric wall. The scan confirmed the attachment of the pseudocyst to the stomach wall. The splenic artery was identified by its pulsation in real-time imaging. The closeness of the splenic artery to this part of the pseudocyst prompted the selection of a cyst entry site that was farther from the artery.

Cyst-wall thickness may be estimated from the ultrasound image. Figure 5-21 shows two sonograms obtained from two different sites of the same pseudocyst. There may be a two to four times difference in wall thickness of the same pseudocyst.

During operations for chronic pancreatitis, evaluation of duct size and location may be accomplished by ultrasound scanning. Figure 5-22 is a sonogram showing pancreatic duct dilation. The pancreatic ducts show both fusiform and saccular dilation. Some of the dilated ducts are 15 millimeters in diameter. Figure 5-23 is an operative pancreatogram of the same gland seen in the previous figure. This pancreatogram confirmed the typical chain-of-lakes dilation of the pancreatic ducts seen in chronic pancreatitis.

Figure 5-24 is a sonogram obtained during another operation for chronic pancreatitis. The gland substance is more echogenic than normal, and the fine reticular pattern of small pancreatic ducts is absent. There are no dilated ducts. Several slit-like, narrow spaces are seen and may represent obliterated ducts. Dissection of this gland during the operation revealed that the gland substance was densely fibrotic. The main pancreatic duct varied from 2 to 5 millimeters in diameter and contained inspissated deposits and some calculi but no dilated ducts.

RESULTS

The results of employing ultrasonography during pancreatic surgery have identified specific applications that we have found helpful in this type of operation. The results are based on the first 42 patients to undergo ultrasonic

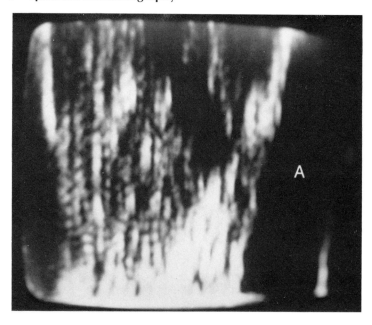

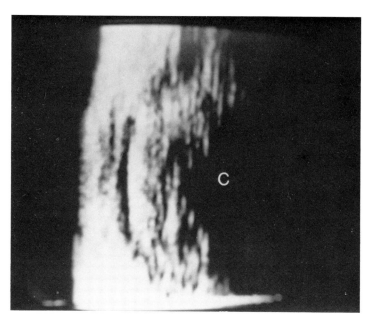

Fig. 5–18. A composite of two sonograms taken at the same operation. The upper sonogram shows internal echoes resulting from inflammatory swelling of the gland immediately superficial to the superior mesenteric artery (A) but no cystic cavity. The lower sonogram reveals the pseudocyst between the body and tail of the gland with a distinct cyst wall and sonolucent cavity (C).

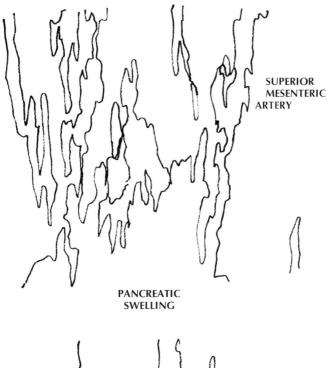

SUPERIOR
MESENTERIC
ARTERY

PANCREATIC
SWELLING

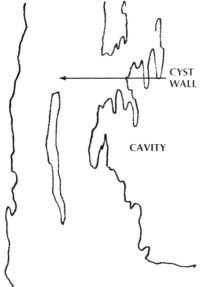

CYST
WALL

CAVITY

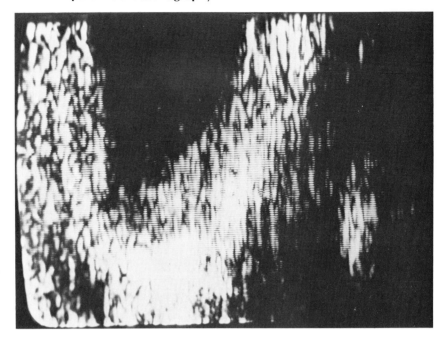

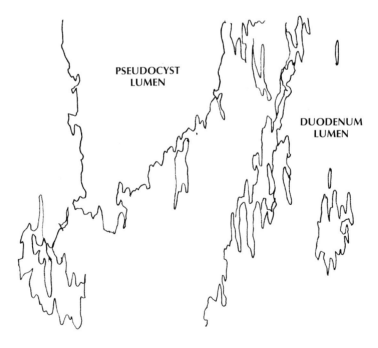

PSEUDOCYST
LUMEN

DUODENUM
LUMEN

Fig. 5–19. Sonogram through a pseudocyst in the head of the pancreas in close proximity to the duodenum.

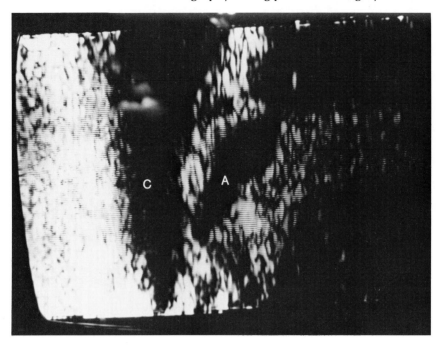

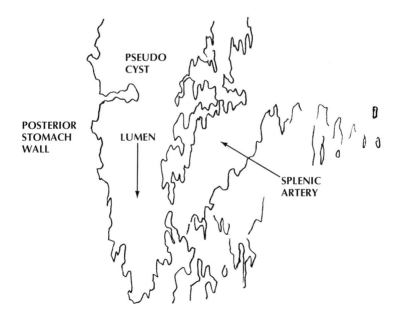

Fig. 5–20. Sonogram of a pancreatic pseudocyst scanned through the posterior wall of the stomach. The edge of the cystic cavity (C) is close to the splenic artery (A), which was seen to pulsate in real-time imaging.

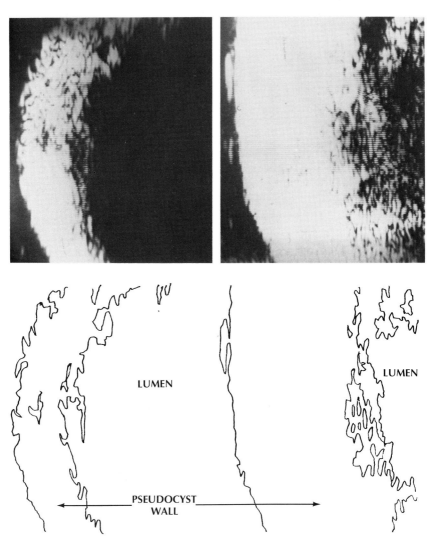

Fig. 5–21. Composite of two sonograms showing different wall thicknesses at two different sites on the same pseudocyst. (Reproduced from Sigel, B: Ultrasonic imaging during biliary and pancreatic surgery. Am J Surg, *141*:84, 1981.)

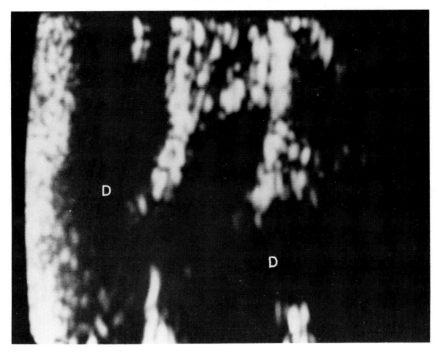

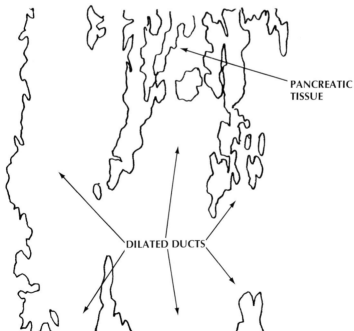

Fig. 5–22.   Sonogram showing dilation of pancreatic ducts (D). (Reproduced from Sigel, B: Ultrasonic imaging during biliary and pancreatic surgery. Am J Surg, *141*:84, 1981.)

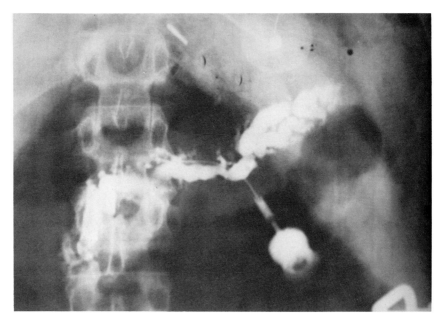

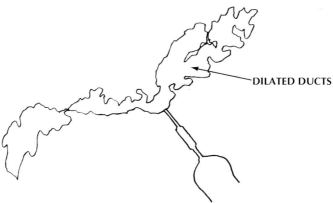

DILATED DUCTS

Fig. 5–23. Operative pancreatogram showing the duct dilation seen in the sonogram in Figure 5–22. (Reproduced from Sigel, B: Ultrasonic imaging during biliary and pancreatic surgery. Am J Surg, *141*:84, 1981.)

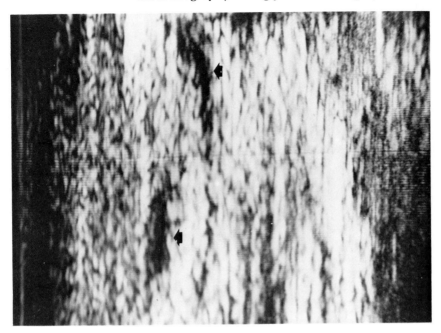

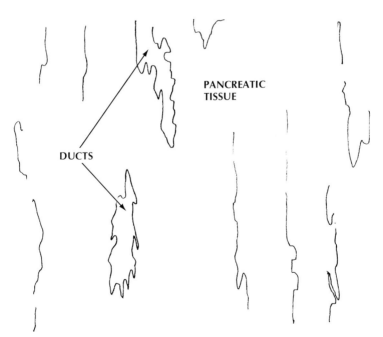

Fig. 5–24. Sonogram of a chronic pancreatitis shows tissue of increased echogenicity surrounding small sonolucent spaces (arrows) that presumably represent compressed or obliterated ducts.

scanning of the pancreas during operation. Of these, 5 patients had a normal pancreas, 10 had a tumor, and the remainder had pancreatitis or its complications.

The ultrasonic examination of the pancreas may be quickly performed with no additional dissection or tissue manipulation than is usually required to expose the gland. A normal pancreas appears ultrasonically as moderately echogenic parenchymal tissue through which a network of fine sonolucent ducts is interspersed. This normal reticular duct structure is often disturbed in tumors of the pancreas as well as in pancreatitis. The splenic and superior mesenteric vessels can usually be observed in close contact with the posterior surface of the gland.

Nine of the ten patients with tumor had lesions in the pancreatic head or periampullary region and were jaundiced. Ultrasonography during surgery was evaluated in terms of providing the following information or assistance in these patients: evaluation of bile duct caliber, exclusion of biliary calculi, patterns of common duct obstruction, status of pancreatic ducts, recognition of tumor tissue, venous invasion, and ultrasound guidance for needle biopsy.

Evaluation of the bile duct caliber by operative ultrasonography has permitted an accurate assessment of duct dilation. In one of the patients with metastasis, ultrasonography revealed that the common hepatic and cystic ducts were dilated, whereas the common bile duct was of a relatively normal caliber. This finding was confirmed by dissection and prompted the selection of a palliative cholecystoenterostomy instead of a choledochoduodenostomy.

Biliary calculi were excluded by ultrasonography early in the course of operation in each patient with tumor. Although the presence of tumor was obvious or highly suspicious in most instances, the presence of calculi in these patients was difficult to exclude on the basis of palpatory findings alone because of the distension and dilation of the gallbladder and bile ducts. Furthermore, in four of the patients, the diagnosis of tumor was not apparent at the initial exploration. The failure to find stones by ultrasound scanning helped to establish more quickly the diagnosis of tumor in these patients.

Tumor obstruction of the distal common bile duct has characteristic image patterns that may be determined by operative ultrasonography. Two patterns have been noted: tapered narrowing above the site of the normal narrowing produced by the sphincter of Oddi and the tumor shelf deformity. The former abnormality is caused by extrinsic compression of the common duct by tumor, whereas the latter is the result of direct infiltration by tumor.

Pancreatic tumors may produce pancreatic duct dilation detectable by operative ultrasonography. This dilation was seen in 8 of the 10 patients with pancreatic or periampullary tumors. In one instance in which pancreatic duct dilation was not observed, the lesion proved to be a relatively small periampullary tumor. This was the only tumor that was resectable. The remaining patients had palliative bypass procedures performed. The normal reticular pattern of fine sonolucent pancreatic ducts in the abnormal glands was replaced by diffuse duct dilation that varied from 5 to 10 millimeters in caliber. The dilation was found throughout the glands and was not limited to the regions near the tumor.

The ultrasonic appearance of a pancreatic tumor is not unique in echogenic properties. In 2 of the 10 patients, tumor tissue appeared to be more echogenic than the remainder of the gland. In the other patients, differences in echogenic properties could not be detected between the tumor region and the seemingly noninvolved portions of the pancreas.

Venous compression by tumor was observed by operative ultrasound scanning in two patients. In both patients, the superior mesenteric-portal vein axis was involved. During ultrasonic imaging, neither vein fluctuated in caliber with respiration and both appeared to be narrowed.

Pancreatic needle biopsy under ultrasonic guidance was performed on two occasions. In one instance, the biopsy established the diagnosis of carcinoma. In the other, the biopsy helped to exclude tumor in what was determined to be pancreatitis limited mostly to the head of the gland. There were no complications following these biopsies.

Of the 27 patients with pancreatitis or its complications, operative ultrasound had the following influence on management. Fourteen patients had pancreatic pseudocysts and one had a pancreatic abscess. In five of the pseudocyst patients and in the abscess patient, drainage procedures were performed on the basis of preoperative information and operative findings. In these six patients, operative ultrasound did not significantly affect management except to corroborate the presence of the lesions. In eight patients, ultrasound provided definitive assistance. During five operations, the location of the pseudocyst was already known and ultrasound helped to select a site for drainage. During three operations, the diagnosis of pseudocyst was first made with certainty by operative ultrasound, which also helped in selecting the site for drainage.

During operation, eight patients were found to have chronic pancreatitis. Our preferred surgical treatment for this condition is to perform a pancreaticoenterostomy (Puestow operation) if the clinical condition warrants intervention and if dilated ducts can be demonstrated. In one patient, preoperative studies and operative findings alone were used to perform a drainage operation. At this operation, equipment failure prevented use of ultrasound to help to locate the dilated duct. In three patients, dilated ducts were recognized preoperatively, and operative ultrasound helped to locate the dilated duct. In one patient, the diagnosis of dilated ducts was made by operative ultrasound because preoperative endoscopic retrograde pancreatography was unsuccessful. In one patient in whom preoperative endoscopic retrograde pancreatography indicated a slightly dilated ductal system, operative ultrasound failed to demonstrate duct dilation. Absence of dilation was confirmed by dissection, and a subtotal pancreatectomy was per-

formed. In two patients, pancreatic duct dilation was discovered by ultrasound, but no pancreatic procedures were performed.

During five operations in which inflammatory abnormalities of the pancreas were found, ultrasound ruled out the presence of pseudocysts or
dilated pancreatic ducts.

Confirmation of an abscess or cystic cavity demonstrated by operative
ultrasound scanning was corroborated in all instances by the operative
findings. Conversely, ultrasonography was able to distinguish masses that
did not contain fluid accumulations. Early in our experience, needle aspiration was attempted to prove the absence of fluid loculations in enlargements
of the pancreas or surrounding tissue after negative ultrasonography. Of 10
such needle aspirations, all were negative. We have since accepted negative
ultrasonic findings as indicative of inflammatory swelling and have stopped
doing exploratory needle aspirations. Thus, operative ultrasound in the
confirmation of abscesses and pseudocysts has been useful in two ways:
verification and exclusion. Verification has been particularly important in
pseudocysts that were small and deep seated. The ability to exclude fluid
loculations in tissue enlargements has reduced exploratory surgical dissection. None of the patients with abscesses or pseudocysts had unnecessary
incisions made into tissue swellings that did not contain fluid collections
requiring drainage.

Once an abscess or pseudocyst cavity has been found, their exact localization at operation is the next step in detection. Although preoperative
ultrasonography or computerized tomography may have indicated the diagnosis and likely site, operative ultrasound has made it possible to localize
precisely a fluid collection in reference to visible landmarks in the operative
field. This ability has been particularly important for small pseudocysts that
may be deep within the pancreas. Localization has consisted not only of
determining the exact site of the abscess or pseudocyst, but also of helping
to estimate its size and extension.

Once an abscess or pseudocyst has been confirmed and localized, operative ultrasound can provide additional information about adjacent structures. Because of anatomic distortion and inflammation, the relation of
important structures, such as the duodenum and the superior mesenteric and
splenic vessels, may not be readily apparent.

In surgery for pseudocyst, advanced knowledge about the thickness of the
pseudocyst wall at several locations has helped in selecting the site of cyst
drainage. Operative ultrasound estimates of cyst-wall thickness have been
within 1 to 3 millimeters of the actual wall thickness observed after cyst
entry.

In our experience in the management of pancreatic abscess and pseudocysts, the various uses of operative ultrasonography—confirmation and localization, recognition of adjacent structures, and estimation of cyst-wall
thickness—all were important factors in helping to decide whether to drain
an area of enlargement. Once this decision was made, ultrasound helped to

decide more precisely where to enter an abscess or pseudocyst for the purpose of establishing drainage.

CONCLUSIONS

Operative ultrasonography may be applied in tumor surgery and in operations for the complications of pancreatitis.

In surgery for pancreatic and periampullary tumors producing common duct obstruction, operative ultrasonography has been helpful in three ways: (1) in providing an accurate measure of common duct dilation; (2) in excluding the presence of obstructing stones in the distal common duct; and (3) in demonstrating patterns of common duct obstruction that were characteristic of extrinsic or intrinsic ductal involvement by tumor.

Operative ultrasonography has not been able to identify tumors on the basis of tissue image characteristics. Two of the tumors showed increased echogenicity. However, chronic pancreatitis also produced tissue with increased echogenicity. Although our experience is still limited, reflective ultrasonography at the frequencies used may not be able to distinguish tumor from inflamed or even normal tissue. Further experience with this type of appraisal is needed.

Operative ultrasound scanning has revealed pancreatic duct dilation in most glands with tumor. This finding reaffirms the risk of pancreatic biopsy for tumor. When a dilated duct is punctured and the obstruction remains unrelieved because the tumor cannot be resected, a pancreatic leak would be more likely to persist, thereby leading to abscess, peritonitis, or fistula formation. Therefore, if pancreatic biopsy is considered advisable, risk may be reduced by performing a needle biopsy under ultrasonic guidance. By use of such control, the possibility of inadvertent puncture of a dilated pancreatic duct may be minimized.

In surgery for the complications of pancreatitis, operative ultrasound has been helpful in the management of pancreatic abscess, pseudocyst, and in chronic pancreatitis.

During an operation for either abscess or pseudocyst, operative ultrasonography accurately confirmed the presence of a fluid loculation in a pancreatic or extrapancreatic enlargement. The converse also applied. Operative ultrasonography may reliably identify the absence of a fluid collection in a pancreatic or extrapancreatic mass or swelling by demonstrating internal echoes consistent with inflammatory edema.

Adjacent structures, such as the duodenum and superior mesenteric and splenic vessels, may be identified by ultrasound scanning during surgery for abscess or pseudocyst. Because these structures may be obscured by distorted anatomy and by inflammation, special care must be given to avoid their injury during dissection and especially during entry into an abscess or cyst cavity to establish drainage. Ultrasonography at the site of anticipated drainage is a useful safeguard to help to prevent such accidents.

At operation for pancreatic pseudocyst, ultrasonography provides an accurate estimate of cyst-wall thickness at various portions of the pseudocyst wall. Wall thickness may vary by a factor of two to four times in the same pseudocyst. The ability to estimate wall thickness prior to entry into a pseudocyst has helped to identify a site with the optimal wall thickness for placement of sutures in the cyst-to-gastrointestinal anastomosis used for drainage.

The combined information provided by operative ultrasound regarding pancreatic abscesses and pseudocysts in terms of confirmation, localization, recognition of adjacent structures to be avoided, and thickness of the cyst wall has assisted the surgeon in making decisions about drainage. Usually, the surgeon must decide not only whether to drain but also where to drain. Questions dealing with the composition of pancreatic or extrapancreatic enlargements and tissue swellings were quickly answered by the ultrasonic demonstration of the presence or absence of fluid loculations. The accuracy of ultrasound in providing information about fluid collections during an operation is high, and this has improved the accuracy of drainage site selection.

During an operation for chronic pancreatitis, ultrasound was useful in helping to decide which surgical procedure to perform. Confirmation of the presence of dilated pancreatic ducts indicated the feasibility of an internal drainage operation. On the other hand, failure to demonstrate dilated pancreatic ducts supported a decision to perform a subtotal pancreatectomy. When dilated pancreatic ducts were present and a decision to perform an internal drainage procedure had been made, ultrasound was employed to guide the passage of an aspirating needle into the main pancreatic duct to facilitate its localization and entry.

RECOMMENDED APPLICATIONS

1. Operative ultrasound may assist in establishing the diagnosis of pancreatic and periampullary tumors that produce common bile duct obstruction. This diagnosis is based mainly on the demonstration of three features:
   A. Dilation of the extrahepatic biliary tract.
   B. Absence of calculi in the common bile duct.
   C. Characteristic appearance of extra and intraductal obstruction by tumor.

If these features are clearly established and visual or palpatory evidence of a mass exists, a working diagnosis of tumor may be made and appropriate operative maneuvers consistent with this diagnosis may be undertaken. This should significantly shorten the decision time in establishing a diagnosis and should avoid unnecessary dissection, cholangiography and, possibly pancreatic biopsy. Cattell and Warren advocated the performance of pancreatectomy for suspected tumor without preliminary biopsy when either the common duct or the pancreatic ducts could be shown to be dilated.[11] Operative ultrasound may provide this information in a more objective manner than inspection and palpation and may expedite the decision process.

When pancreatic biopsy is considered essential, it may be more safely performed under ultrasonic control. By guiding a biopsy needle directly into the pancreas or, preferably, into the pancreas through the duodenum, ultrasound may help to avoid inadvertent puncture of major blood vessels and pancreatic ducts, which are usually dilated when in association with tumors producing common duct obstruction.

2. Operative ultrasound may provide information during surgery for pancreatic abscess and pseudocyst. This information may include the following factors:

A. Confirmation of a fluid loculation within a pancreatic or extrapancreatic mass or swelling.

B. Specific localization of abscesses and pseudocysts in relation to identifiable anatomic landmarks seen at operation.

C. Discovery of difficult-to-recognize adjacent structures that should be protected from injury during dissection and performance of a drainage procedure.

D. Estimation of the thickness of the wall of a pancreatic pseudocyst at various locations.

Such information may be helpful in two respects. First, a determination may be made regarding the existence of an abscess or pseudocyst cavity. This is important not only when fluid loculations are present, but also when ruling out fluid collections in pancreatic and extra-pancreatic masses and enlargements produced by inflammatory edema. This determination and the additional information regarding adjacent structures and wall thickness of cysts may aid the surgeon in a second respect: selecting the most appropriate site for entry into an abscess or pseudocyst cavity for the purpose of establishing drainage.

3. Operative ultrasonography may help in surgery for chronic pancreatitis by:

A. Confirming the presence of dilated pancreatic ducts.

B. Localizing dilated pancreatic ducts for internal drainage operations.

Confirmation of the presence of dilated pancreatic ducts indicates the feasibility of performing an internal drainage procedure between the dilated ducts and the intestinal tract. The absence of pancreatic duct dilation supports a decision to perform a different operation, such as partial or subtotal excision of the gland. When the pancreatic ducts are dilated, ultrasonography permits their quick and precise localization for entry and drainage.

CHAPTER **6**

ULTRASONOGRAPHY DURING RENAL SURGERY

The use of ultrasound during surgical procedures was first employed in operations for renal calculi. A report by Schlegel and associates appeared in 1961 and described the authors' experience with A-mode ultrasound scanning during operation for nephrolithiasis.[12] Although they reported success in localization, this technique did not become popular, probably because of the difficulty in interpreting one-dimensional images. The A-mode spikes representing the increased echogenicity produced by the renal calculi had to be distinguished from spikes of increased amplitude produced by fibrosis or the interface between renal and fatty tissue. Real-time B-mode ultrasound scanning of the kidney during surgery was first described by Cook and Lytton, and this technique has overcome some of the problems of A-mode imaging.[13,14]

The principal use of imaging ultrasound during renal surgery is to confirm and localize renal calculi to facilitate their extraction. In this chapter, the utilization of ultrasonography during nephrolithotomy is considered in terms of rationale, technique, and findings. The results of this operative diagnostic procedure are presented. From this, conclusions are reached and recommendations are made for how this particular type of operative ultrasonography can be best applied in renal surgery.

ULTRASONOGRAPHY DURING NEPHROLITHOTOMY

Renal surgery for stones is never attempted without preoperative imaging studies that indicate the size, number, and location of the calculi. Despite this information, the exact localization and removal of stones during an operation may present problems that can prolong dissection and operating time, increase parenchymal kidney damage, and result in retention of renal stones or stone fragments. Cook and Lytton have reviewed this problem and have summarized the various measures used to assist the surgeon. Such measures include radiography, nephroscopy, and use of plasma coagulum to entrap small stone fragments. These workers selected operative ultrasound scanning as the preferable means for operative localization because it provided a three-dimensional sense to the location of stones as the scanning probe is manipulated over the entire exposed surface of the kidney parenchyma and pelvis.[14]

We found three main indications for using imaging ultrasound during surgery for renal lithiasis.[15] The first was to confirm and locate stones in the surgically exposed kidney prior to pyelotomy or nephrotomy. This was particularly useful for small stones that may have shifted position. The second indication was to provide guidance for an exploratory needle directed to the stone. This was usually done for small stones that were in a fixed position within a calyx or an intrarenal pelvis and that required an incision through renal tissue to be extracted. A small nephrotomy directly over the stone produced the least damage. Finally, ultrasound was employed after stone extraction as a check to insure that all calculi had been removed.

Technique

After the kidney has been exposed and palpated, the ultrasound examination should be performed over the entire accessible surface of the organ, including the posterior and anterior aspect of the kidney. The pelvis, if in its normal extrarenal position, should also be scanned.

The kidney should be maintained in as normal a position as will allow passage of the transducer-probe over its surface. Usually, the kidney may be kept in a relatively deep position within the operative field. This position more readily permits the kidney to be submerged after saline is introduced into the operative field. The transducer-probe should be positioned in "dry placement" over the deepest aspect of the kidney or renal pelvis (Fig. 6-1). The scan paths should begin deep and progress to more superficial aspects of the kidney. When over the pelvis, an acoustic window of 5 to 10 mm should be maintained. When over the kidney substance, this distance can be reduced, but the tip of the probe should be maintained a few millimeters off the surface of the organ (Fig. 6-2).

After introduction of warm saline, the kidney is scanned. If probe motion is restricted in the depth of the operative field, transverse and longitudinal angulation may be the most practical maneuvers. The transducer-probe

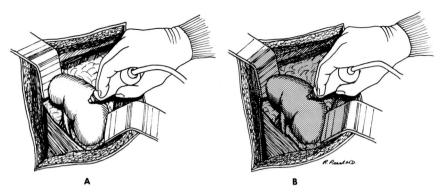

Fig. 6–1. *A,* "Dry placement" of the transducer-probe in the operative field. This positioning of the transducer-probe over the kidney is done before the introduction of saline to be certain of the location and orientation of the probe in reference to the kidney. *B,* The operative field is immersed in saline during scanning.

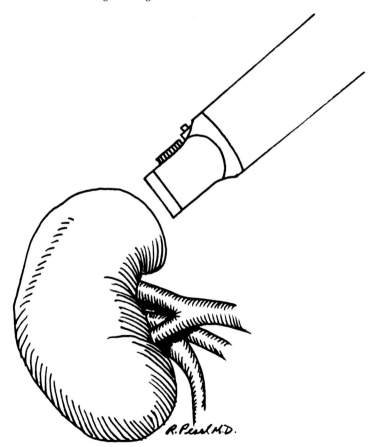

Fig. 6–2. Illustration of an ultrasound scan of the kidney. The transducer-probe is kept a few millimeters from the kidney to maintain an acoustic window.

should then be positioned more superficially in the operative field. The preferred maneuver is longitudinal scanning, which should be performed with transverse angulation over the entire posterior and anterior surface of the kidney.

After the stone or stones have been identified, the surgeon must decide which approach to use to gain entry into the drainage system. The decision usually involves whether to open the pelvis or to go directly through renal tissue. Whenever possible, a pelvic incision is preferred. However, if a stone is known to be in a calyx and not accessible through the pelvis, or if the pelvis is surrounded by renal tissue, a nephrotomy incision should be used. Ultrasonic guidance for the passage of an exploratory needle through renal parenchyma to the location of a stone can be provided in two ways: free-hand or with the aid of a needle guide.

With the free-hand method, the stone is visualized by ultrasound, and the position and angle of the transducer-probe to the surface of the kidney is carefully noted. A 25-gauge spinal needle is inserted into the kidney at a point where the plastic window of the transducer was centered. The angle of the needle should duplicate the angle that was assumed by the transducer-probe when the stone was visualized. This technique for needle passage may be used with larger stones (5 mm or more in diameter) that are superficial (about 1 cm or less below the surface).

Smaller stones are best approached with the use of a needle-guide adapter, which comes as an attachment to the High Stoy transducer-probe. With the adapter in place, the stone is first located and its depth is calculated. Depth is estimated on the Bronson-Turner unit and measured directly on the SP-100-B unit using a range indicator. This indicator places concentric lines on the monitor screen at known distances and permits a determination of depth to within 1 or 2 millimeters.

After the depth of the stone is known, the needle guide should be slid to the corresponding depth position mark on the adapter. When the needle point enters the center of the sound beam, this adjustment places the tip of the exploratory needle exactly at the preset distance from the plastic window of the transducer-probe. During this maneuver, the needle must be fixed in the guide groove and in a slot near the end of the transducer-probe to maintain a proper position (Fig. 6-3).

The transducer-probe and attached preset needle guide should be placed against the kidney surface. The stone should be visualized, and the probe should be adjusted to bring the stone image of the monitor equidistant between the upper and lower borders of the monitor screen. With this position held as steadily as possible, a 25-gauge spinal needle should be slotted into the grooves of the probe and needle guide and advanced until the needle echoes are seen on the monitor screen. If all maneuvers are properly performed, the needle should appear on the monitor in close proximity to the stone or even in direct contact with the stone. Direct contact may be associated with a grating sensation of the needle against the calculus.

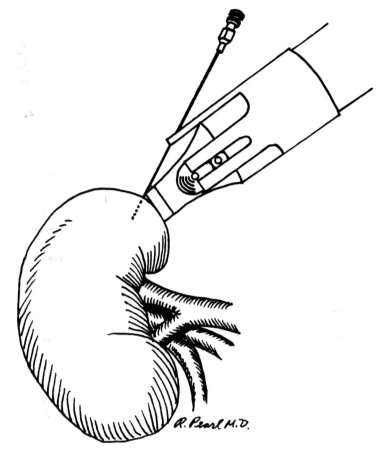

Fig. 6–3. Illustration of ultrasonic guidance of an exploratory needle to the site of a stone using a needle-guide adapter attached to the transducer-probe.

After the needle has been positioned either free-hand or with the needle guide, the needle should be maintained in position while a small incision is made along the needle tract. The length of the incision is determined by the size of the stone and is usually 6 to 15 mm long. The incision should be extended into the calyx. A Kelley hemostat should be inserted through the incision, and the stone should be grasped and removed.

Following the extraction of all stones believed to be present, the operator's finger should be introduced into any pyelotomy or nephrotomy incision of sufficient size to permit digital exploration. All palpated fragments are removed. Ultrasonography should be repeated to make certain that no stones or stone fragments are retained.

Prior to ultrasound examination, warm saline solution is reintroduced into the operative field. This process must entail the injection of saline into the renal pelvis and calyceal system through the pyelotomy and nephrotomy incisions. The introduction of saline solution into the kidney's interior should be performed in a manner that displaces all air within the collecting system. This is accomplished by using a 20- to 50-ml syringe and a 19- or 18-gauge needle. If the collecting system is dilated, a small-caliber, red rubber catheter should be substituted for the needle to provide more rapid filling. The needle or catheter and syringe should be used to deliver a copious amount of saline solution to all recesses within the kidney and pelvis. If possible, the position of the kidney may be manipulated to permit escape of all air bubbles.

Ultrasonography should be repeated in a manner similar to the initial examination. Particular attention should be paid to the regions from which stones were extracted. If any suspicious images are seen, the first course of action should be to irrigate the region to make certain that no air bubbles remain trapped within the collecting system. If echogenic structures remain, further exploration should be performed.

At completion of all ultrasonography, we usually take an operative radiograph of the kidney. This is done to provide maximum assurance that all calculi have been removed.

Findings

The ultrasonic image of a normal kidney is shown in Figure 6-4. This shows the renal cortex and a minor calyx communicating with a major calyx.

Renal calculi were usually markedly echogenic. Most of the reflection was produced by the most superficial layers of the stone. This characteristically produced a narrow, highly intense echogenic image in B-mode scanning associated with a dense acoustic shadow. Figures 6-5, 6-6, and 6-7 show examples of renal calculi scanned during nephrolithotomy surgery.

The features of the ultrasound images are sufficiently different from radiographs to warrant special emphasis to reduce interpretation errors. The mainstay of diagnosis is to identify correctly a discrete area of increased echogenicity and an acoustic shadow emanating from the echogenic area and passing off to the deep margin of the image. Errors arise if either of these features is not clearly identified.

Errors leading to a false-negative interpretation are the result mainly of two situations. The first situation results from missing the characteristic ultrasound features of the stone. This may be caused by decreased echogenicity of the stone, abnormal kidney anatomy producing distracting images, or, most commonly, by a failure to systematically scan the entire renal collecting system. The scanning maneuvers over the kidney must cover the entire organ. A stone also may be missed because it is obscured by an acoustic shadow produced by another structure. The usual situation producing this error is a large stone with a prominent acoustic shadow that hides smaller calculi. The best way to avoid this mistake is to be especially attentive to the presence of small stones in acoustically shaded areas and to

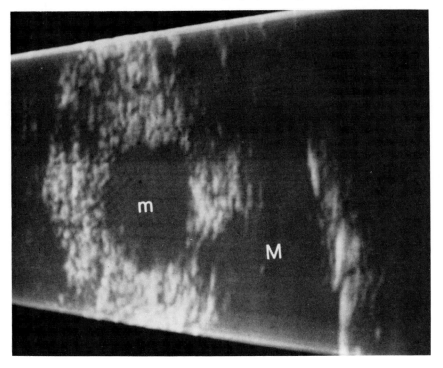

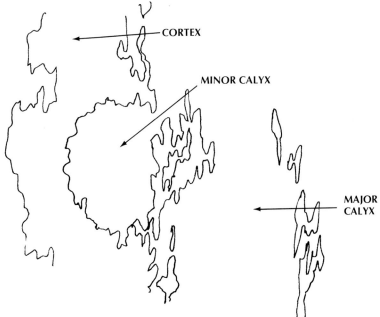

Fig. 6–4. Sonogram of a normal kidney shows renal cortex and a minor calyx (m) communicating with a major calyx (M).

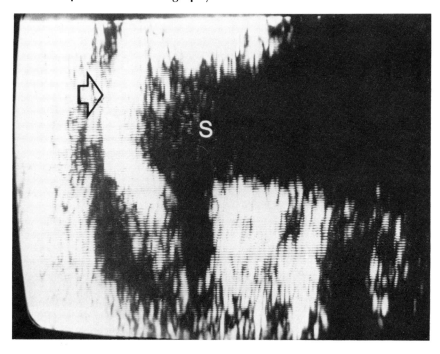

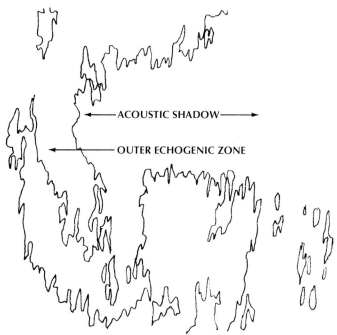

Fig. 6–5. Sonogram of a 3-cm stone within a dilated calyx. The outer zone of the stone (arrow) is highly echogenic. An acoustic shadow (S) passes from the echogenic area to the right margin of the monitor screen.

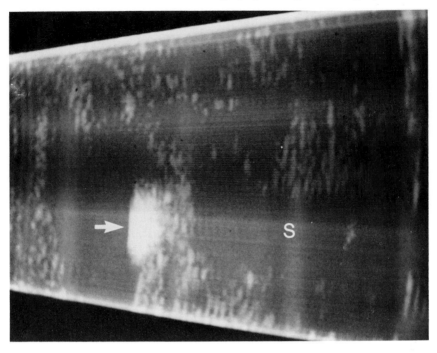

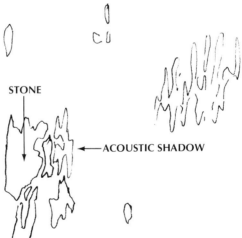

Fig. 6–6. Sonogram of a calyceal stone (arrow) about 3 to 4 mm in diameter. An acoustic shadow (S) is also seen.

scan transversely with the transducer-probe in a manner that ensonifies the region behind the stone.

Errors most likely to cause a false-positive diagnosis of stones are the result of the production of strong echoes from the surface or within the kidney. The source of these echoes is a high acoustic impedance mismatch (see Chap. 1, *The Basics of Ultrasound*), which results from fibrosis or adipose tissue

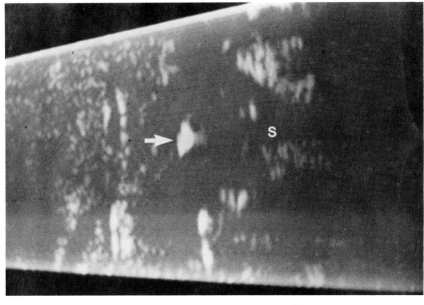

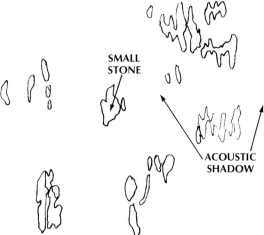

Fig. 6–7. Sonogram of a small calyceal stone (arrow) about 2 to 3 mm in diameter. A thin acoustic shadow (S) is present. (Reproduced from Sigel, B: Ultrasonic scanning during operation for renal calculi. J Urol, in press.)

interfaced with kidney tissue. An important combination of features leading to a false-positive diagnosis of stone is produced by increased fibrosis in the tissue superficial to a calyx. This may produce an echogenic area adjacent to the nonechogenic region of the calyceal cavity. Such a combination of an echogenic area immediately next to the sonolucent zone produced by the calyx may resemble a calculus and its acoustic shadow. This resemblance is particularly likely to occur if the collecting system is dilated. Dilation may extend the region of sonolucency to the deep margin of the monitor view, thereby simulating an acoustic shadow. The best way to avoid this error is to note carefully the configuration and location of the echogenic area. If due to tissue fibrosis, the echogenic area is usually seen outside rather than inside a calyx. In addition, an attempt should be made to trace the extent of the "shadow" to make sure that it is not simply a dilated calyx or pelvis. A simple maneuver may be helpful in proving that a sonolucent area is produced by a calyx and is not an acoustic shadow (Fig. 6-8). This maneuver consists of compressing the kidney gently with the transducer-probe. Compression should reduce the size of the calyceal sonolucent image and may bring the renal parenchyma into view at the far (right) side of the monitor screen. This would tend to rule out an acoustic shadow, which would be expected to extend across the screen and to cut through the tissue image.

Another source for false-positive diagnoses of renal stones is air bubbles. Air bubbles may occur after the collecting system has been opened. A clue to the presence of air bubbles is their tendency to float to the uppermost portion of a cavity. They are also more likely than stones to change position. The best assurance to prevent the imaging of air bubbles or pockets is to be certain that the collecting system is filled with fluid and that an egress is provided for the escape of air bubbles during instillation of saline solution.

RESULTS

We have reported our experience obtained during 16 operations performed to remove stones from the kidney.[15] These results may be summarized as follows.

In one patient operated on early in our experience, ultrasound missed two retained stone fragments after extraction of a staghorn calculus. This was our only false-negative result. There have been no false-positive findings, although we have encountered several instances of renal fibrosis that showed an increase in echogenicity. Our positive results are presented in terms of the primary indications for ultrasonography in renal lithiasis surgery.

The first of these indications was to confirm and localize stones early during operation. This was achieved by ultrasound at nine operations. In one patient operated on for another condition, ultrasound confirmed the absence of stones. In eight patients, ultrasound provided more precise information about existing stones both in terms of their number and their location. At one operation, ultrasound correctly identified a single stone in a patient in whom preoperative studies suggested the presence of three stones.

In another patient, three radiopaque calculi were detected on preoperative studies. During the operation, ultrasound found these calculi and, in addition, discovered that three stones, which were nonopaque on the roentgenogram, were occupying three different minor calyces. All calculi were extracted employing small nephrotomy incisions.

A second indication for operative ultrasound was to guide an exploratory needle to locate precisely intrarenal stones. This procedure was employed

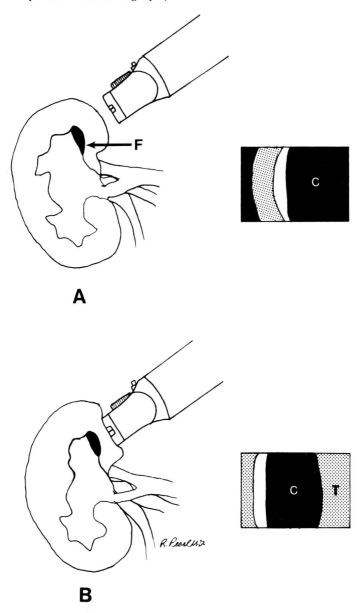

Fig. 6–8. *A,* Illustration of an ultrasound scan shows a fibrosed area of tissue (F) adjacent to a dilated calyx. On the monitor screen, the area of fibrosis is more echogenic (white) than the more superificial kidney tissue. The sonolucent calyx (C) may be mistaken for an acoustic shadow. *B,* Illustration of how this erroneous picture may be clarified. By compressing the kidney and calyx gently with the transducer-probe, the width of the imaged sonolucent calyx is decreased, and deeper renal tissue (T) is seen. This decrease in width would not occur in the presence of a stone because the acoustic shadow would pass to the end of the monitor screen.

during six operations. Ultrasound permitted exact and rapid localization, resulting in relatively small incisions through renal parenchyma and a significant shortening of operating time.

The third indication for using ultrasonography during renal stone surgery was to check the operative site for retained calculi after stone extraction. This was performed at seven operations. Except for the one false-negative result, ultrasound correctly assessed the status of stone removal in six patients. Five of these proved negative, whereas in one patient, four stone fragments were found after removal of a staghorn calculus.

CONCLUSIONS

Operative ultrasonography has proved helpful for each of the indications identified in nephrolithiasis surgery. These were (1) to confirm and localize calculi during an operation in reference to visible anatomic landmarks; (2) to guide an exploratory needle through renal parenchyma to place precisely and minimize the size of nephrotomy incisions; and (3) to survey the operative site after stone extraction to be certain that all calculi had been removed.

Pre-extraction confirmation and localization were important in determining if previously recognized calculi had migrated, if suggestive evidence of stones on preoperative studies could be verified, and if additional stones could be found. The diagnosis of additional stones was particularly significant in the patient in whom nonopaque stones were discovered by operative ultrasound because, without ultrasound, these stones probably would have been missed. This experience parallels that reported for preoperative use of ultrasound for detecting stones that were nonopaque on the roetgenogram. Such stones can only be detected radiographically as filling defects in excretory contrast studies. This type of study would be difficult to obtain during an operation. Operative ultrasound, therefore, may be ideally suited for detecting such calculi.

Ultrasonic guidance of exploratory needles to facilitate the placement of nephrotomy incisions probably has been the most useful function of ultrasound in renal surgery. The use of ultrasound for this purpose has often resulted in smaller nephrotomy incisions and in search times lasting only a few minutes. We believe that ultrasound not only has contributed to less dissection and shortened operating time, but also has led to a higher stone retrieval rate.

Postextraction surveillance with ultrasound has the potential for reducing postextraction operative radiography. We have performed radiography prior to closure as a final check to make certain that all stones have been removed. By using ultrasound first in this surveillance, retained stone fragments have been found and removed. This has reduced the number of radiographs needed to show that the operative site has been totally cleared of stones.

RECOMMENDED APPLICATION

Based on our experience, we would recommend the following course of action in employing real-time B-mode ultrasound scanning during operations for nephrolithiasis.

There are three principal indications for the use of ultrasound in this type of surgery: initial scanning to confirm and locate calculi, guidance of exploratory needles in situations in which nephrotomy incisions are contemplated, and, following stone extraction, making certain that all calculi have been removed.

1. Initial scanning should be performed as soon as the kidney is exposed. The posterior and anterior surfaces of the kidney and the renal pelvis should be systemically examined.

2. After all calculi have been identified, a decision regarding the site of entry to remove the stones must be made. A pyelotomy incision should be used for pelvic stones or calculi that may be extracted through the pelvis. For stones fixed within minor calyces or when the pelvis is intrarenal and surrounded by renal parenchyma, an incision through renal tissue is needed. In this circumstance, ultrasound may be helpful in permitting the use of small incisions placed directly over the calculi. The approach for such stone extraction consists of the following steps:

   A. Ultrasonic guidance is used to pass an exploratory needle to the site of the calculus. This may be done free-hand for larger stones or with the use of a needle guide attached to the transducer-probe for smaller stones.

   B. Once the needle is imaged in proximity to the calculus, a small incision through renal parenchyma is made just large enough to extract the stone. This process may be repeated elsewhere in the kidney if multiple stones are present.

Ultrasonic assistance for stone extraction reduces tissue dissection and operating time and should result in fewer stones being retained.

3. Following stone extraction and prior to closure of any nephrotomy or pyelotomy incisions, the kidney should be scanned again to make certain that all stone fragments have been removed. After this examination, a final radiograph should be taken to document that the operative field has been cleared of all calculi.

CHAPTER 7

ULTRASONOGRAPHY DURING VASCULAR SURGERY

Operative ultrasound may assist the surgeon performing vascular recon-struction. Two operative applications of imaging ultrasound have been evaluated and may be clinically useful.[16] One use provides additional information to that already determined from the preoperative arteriography. This enables ultrasound to play a supplementary role to arteriography. The use of this technique to assess segments of vessels exposed during operation and about which previous arteriography did not provide complete informa-tion could potentially reduce the need for operative arteriography. A second application employs ultrasound to determine whether vascular defects, such as strictures, thrombi, or intimal flaps, have inadvertently been left behind after vascular reconstruction.

The application of operative ultrasound to assess segments of exposed arteries for atherosclerotic disease was an extension of previously developed technology in noninvasive imaging.[17] High-frequency B-mode has been used transcutaneously to detect and quantitate atherosclerotic plaques. Thus, the feasibility of this approach has been established and it is possible to consider operative evaluation.

The use of operative ultrasound to detect vascular defects immediately after surgery did not have established precedents derived from previous experience with ultrasound. Consequently, to establish a basis for clinical application and to obtain some indication of the accuracy of this approach, animal experimentation was needed.

This chapter summarizes first the results of animal experiments that were performed to demonstrate the feasibility of operative ultrasound to detect

135

vascular defects. The utilization of this approach in vascular surgery is considered in terms of indications, technique, and findings. Results are presented from which conclusions are drawn, and recommendations are made for the use of operative ultrasonography during vascular surgery.

EXPERIMENTAL BACKGROUND FOR DETECTION OF VASCULAR DEFECTS

Two experimental studies were performed to determine the feasibility of operative ultrasonography in the detection of vascular defects resulting from operation. In each study, defects were created in the aorta of dogs to simulate lesions that might occur during operation.

Experiments to determine the type and size of lesions detectable by ultrasound.[18] In this study, four types of defects were established. These were strictures, thrombi, subintimal hematomas, and intimal flaps. Real-time B-mode scanning was performed directly on exposed blood vessels. The size of each lesion was varied to provide an indication of the minimal size that would be detectable by ultrasound. Relatively small strictures (diameter reductions by 25%), thrombi, and subintimal hematomas could be imaged. Intimal flaps were varied in size from 1 to 5 millimeters of undermining. Ultrasound was able to detect 68% of the 1-millimeter flaps and 100% of the flaps that were 2 millimeters or larger.

Experimental comparison of arteriography and ultrasonography in detecting vascular defects.[19] In this evaluation, 25% diameter strictures, small thrombi, and intimal flaps (either 2 or 5 millimeters in size) were examined by portable arteriography (one anterior-posterior view), serial biplane arteriography, and real-time B-mode ultrasound scanning. All three diagnostic procedures showed high specificity. The sensitivity of all three techniques was relatively good and comparable in diagnosing strictures. Serial biplane arteriography was superior to portable arteriography in the detection of intimal flaps and thrombi. However, ultrasound proved to be significantly more sensitive than serial biplane arteriography in the identification of intimal flaps and thrombi.

The conclusions from these experiments were that real-time high resolution B-mode ultrasound imaging in direct contact with exposed blood vessels was a sensitive and specific diagnostic technique for detecting strictures, thrombi, subintimal hematomas, and intimal flaps. The studies indicated the feasibility for the use of operative real-time ultrasound imaging to detect vascular defects following vascular reconstructive surgery.

UTILIZATION OF ULTRASONOGRAPHY DURING VASCULAR SURGERY

The use of real-time ultrasonic imaging during vascular surgery has evolved in relation to the specific requirements of the operative procedures. In this section, the principal indications for the use of imaging ultrasound during vascular surgery are reviewed, the technique is described, and characteristic findings are presented.

Indications

There are two main reasons for using real-time B-mode scanning during vascular surgery: to evaluate the presence and extent of atherosclerotic disease in arteries exposed at operation and to detect vascular defects immediately after vascular reconstruction.

The use of operative ultrasound during an operation to assess arteries for atherosclerotic disease is a role that is secondary and complementary to the use of preoperative arteriography. Arteriography is a prerequisite to surgery not only to confirm the presence of significant disease, but also to provide assurance that vascular reconstruction is possible. Thus, the status of the arteries is usually well known prior to operation. At times, because of incomplete filling with contrast material, arteriography may not be able to demonstrate the exact extent of occlusive disease. In other circumstances, arteriography may be complete, but the surgeon may still have difficulty in locating a particular arterial segment because of limited operative exposure. In these situations, ultrasound may help in the selection of a site to enter an artery and may reduce the need to expose long segments of the vessel for purposes of identification. Operative ultrasound may help to assess quickly exposed blood vessels and to make decisions about the most appropriate surgical management.

The use of imaging ultrasound to detect vascular defects immediately after reconstructive surgery and prior to closure of the operative incision is the other prime indication for using real-time B-mode ultrasonography during vascular surgery. Ultrasonic scanning should be performed after clamps have been removed and blood flow restored following endarterectomy or anastomosis. Areas that have undergone operative manipulation should be carefully surveyed, employing multiple sections to detect evidence of strictures, thrombi, or intimal flaps. This examination should include segments that have been directly visualized, segments that have not been directly exposed but have been blindly endarterectomized, and vessel sites that have been compressed by vascular clamps.

Technique

Operative ultrasound may be performed at any time during surgery to evaluate arterial segments for atherosclerotic disease. Usually, if this is needed, these examinations are conducted prior to arterial clamping and entry.

The technique for evaluating arterial segments for disease consists of positioning the transducer-probe in "dry placement" in a longitudinal orientation and maintaining a distance of about 5 mm from the surface of the vessel. Warm saline is introduced to provide acoustic coupling. Often, the vessel is superficially situated in the operative field, thereby preventing its submergence beneath the saline. In these circumstances, the edges of the operative wound should be retracted upward to deepen the operative field and to create a trough that would permit the saline to cover the vessels completely (Fig. 7-1).

The principal maneuver for ultrasonic examination to detect disease is longitudinal scanning with transverse angulation. This should be conducted im multiple planes to allow visualization of a number of sections to obtain a three-dimensional survey of the vessel.

Once an abnormal vascular segment is recognized, a special variation of transverse scanning should be performed. This maneuver is termed arcing and consists of transverse scanning with a change in the position of the transducer-probe axis to keep the transducer-probe pointed toward the center of the blood vessel (Fig. 7-2). This maneuver is limited by the exposure of the vessel. However, its performance, even to a limited extent, may provide valuable three-dimensional information about an abnormality within the vessel.

The ultrasonic examination for vascular defects immediately after reconstruction varies according to the type of operative procedure performed.

Following endarterectomy, ultrasound scanning is similar to examining an artery for atheromatous disease (Fig. 7-3). The transducer-probe scanning maneuvers consist of longitudinal scanning with transverse angulation along

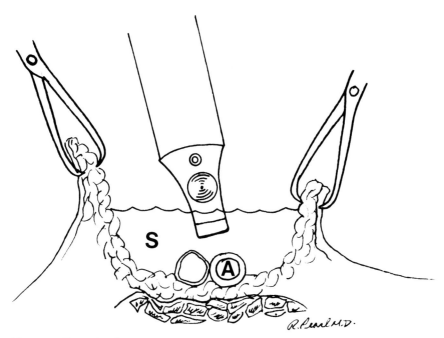

Fig. 7–1. Illustration showing a cross section of an operative wound in which the artery (A) is in a superficial position. The skin flaps have been retracted upward to produce a trough that permits saline (S) to cover the vessel completely.

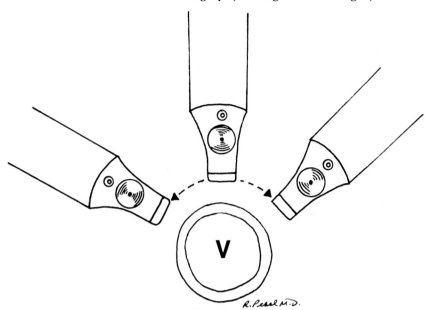

Fig. 7–2. Illustration showing a vessel (V) in cross section that is undergoing transverse scanning. During this maneuver, the transducer-probe position is changed to keep the transducer-probe axis pointed toward the center of the vessel. This variation of transverse scanning is termed arcing.

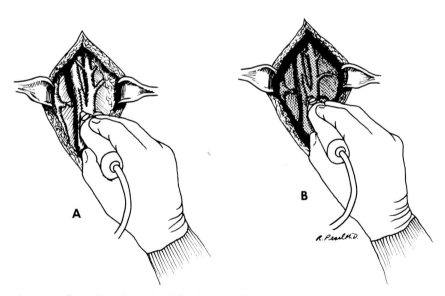

Fig. 7–3. Illustration of scanning following carotid endarterectomy. A, "Dry" placement of the transducer. B, Scanning maneuvers after the addition of saline.

parallel scan paths. These scan paths traverse all vascular segments that were involved in operative manipulation. Care is taken to maintain the transducer probe at least 5 mm away from the vessel surface. Any abnormal findings should be re-examined both by longitudinal and arcing scan maneuvers.

Following end-to-end anastomosis, scanning maneuvers similar to those used following endarterectomy are employed.

Ultrasonic examination following end-to-side anastomosis is more complex because three vascular segments come together at the anastomosis. The objectives of the examination are to visualize the entire circumference of the anastomosis and to survey all areas submitted to operative manipulation. The vast majority of end-to-side anastomoses are performed to bypass occluded arteries employing either synthetic or autogenous vein grafts. These bypass grafts usually run parallel to the native occluded arteries. Consequently, the anastomoses are performed at an acute angle, and the grafts often cover a portion of the native arteries that comprise a part of the anastomoses.

There are two ways to scan end-to-side bypass anastomoses in which the grafts may obscure a part of the native arteries: through-the-graft scanning and lateral scanning.

Through-the-graft scanning is performed at the site of anastomosis, and the transducer-probe is passed across the suture line to image the native artery to which the graft is sutured. This approach to scanning the anastomosis is the simplest, and the entire circumference of the junction may be

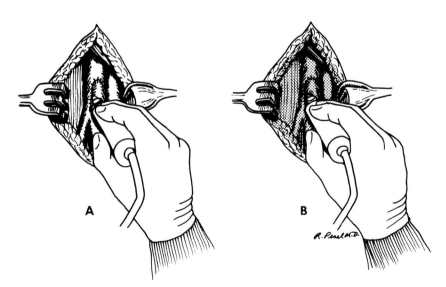

Fig. 7–4. Illustration of scanning of the proximal anastomosis of a bypass graft. *A,* "Dry" placement of the transducer-probe, which employs a through-the-graft scan. *B,* Addition of saline provides acoustic coupling.

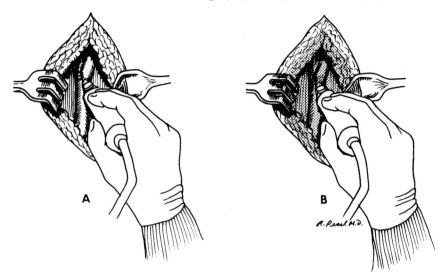

Fig. 7–5. Illustration of scanning of the distal anastomosis through the graft. First the transducer-probe is positioned in dry placement (A), and then saline is added (B).

surveyed (Fig. 7-4 and 7-5). Some synthetic graft material is echogenic and prevents penetration of the ultrasound beam. In these circumstances, the anastomosis must be scanned from its lateral aspect.

Lateral scanning usually is performed from both sides to make certain that the entire circumference of the anastomosis is covered (Fig. 7-6). Particular attention should be given to the parts of the anastomosis that were not sutured under direct vision.

All segments of the vessels that were manipulated in any way should be ultrasonically scanned. This especially applies to the sites where vascular clamps were applied.

Findings

Normal arteries demonstrate echogenic walls and sonolucent lumens (Fig. 7-7). Sonolucent lumens are seen if blood is flowing. If blood flow is obstructed or conditions for stasis exist, unclotted whole blood may demonstrate internal echoes. This has been observed clinically and experimentally (Fig. 7-8). In a series of in vivo and in vitro experiments, we have shown that echogenicity of unclotted blood only occurs with high-resolution ultrasonography at frequencies of 5 MHz and above. In addition, the blood must be static. Our work indicates that the mechanism for this echogenicity is sound reflecting from red-cell aggregation. We have correlated this increased echogenicity with conditions that are known to increase red-cell aggregation, such as increases in hematocrit, fibrinogen, and other macromolecules and increased temperature. We have observed an increase in echogenicity in blood that showed increased rouleaux formation.[20,21]

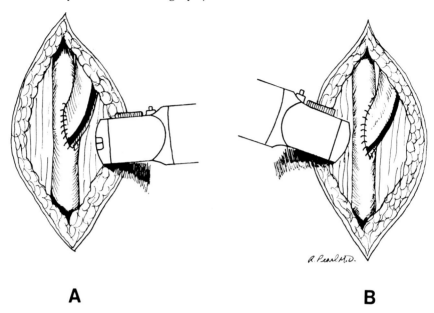

A   **B**

Fig. 7–6. Illustration of lateral scanning of an end-to-side anastomosis. The anastomosis is usually scanned from both sides.

Flowing venous blood detected during experimental surgery in dogs has demonstrated internal echoes moving with the stream. These may represent moving red-cell aggregations. We have occasionally observed such moving internal echoes in jugular vein flow in normal circumstances. However, we have not observed blood echogenicity in fast-moving arterial flow. The clinical significance of these ultrasonic echoes from the lumen of blood vessels is unknown.

The most important clinical abnormalities of vessel walls that may be detected by imaging ultrasound during surgical operations are arteriosclerotic disease and vascular defects resulting from vascular reconstructive surgery. These findings will be presented by considering first the experimental results that demonstrate the ultrasonic appearance of strictures, thrombi, and intimal flaps. Then, the ultrasonic appearance of abnormalities produced by disease and of vascular defects that were associated with reconstructive surgery will be described.

The ultrasonic scans of vascular defects produced in the dog aorta are seen in Figures 7-9, 7-10, 7-11, and 7-12. These scans were produced under circumstances that closely resembled the conditions at operation. Figure 7-9 demonstrates a strictured narrowing of about 25% of the diameter. Figure 7-10 shows a small thrombus. Figure 7-11 depicts multiple views of the same intimal flap recorded in different positions because of motion of the flap in the flow stream. Figure 7-12 shows intimal flaps varying in size from 1 to 5 millimeters.

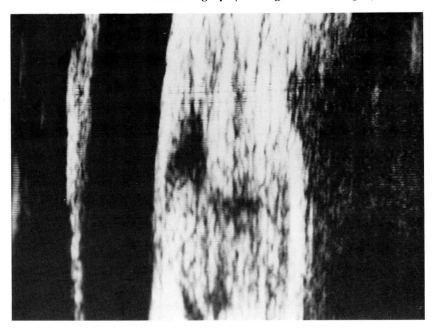

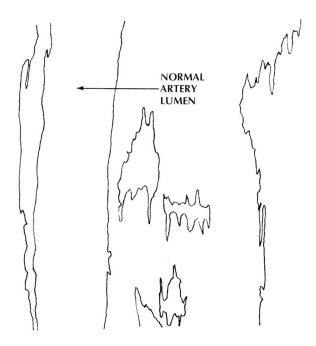

NORMAL
ARTERY
LUMEN

Fig. 7–7. Sonogram of a longitudinal section of a normal artery.

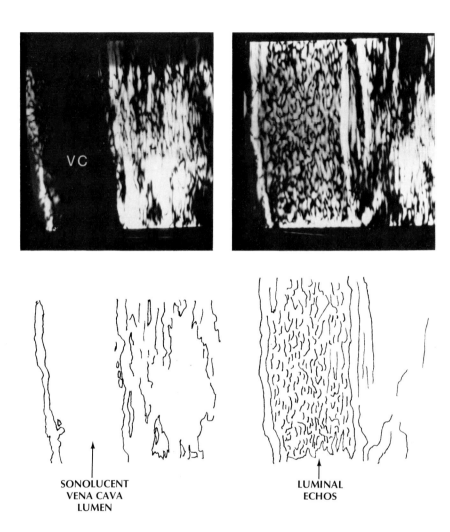

Fig. 7–8. A composite of two sonograms showing echogenicity following blood stasis. The sonogram at left shows an unoccluded inferior vena cava in a dog with a sonolucent lumen. The sonogram on the right shows blood stasis in the same vena cava that has been occluded for 3 minutes by clamps above and below the scanned segment. Numerous internal echoes are produced by aggregation of red cells resulting from the stasis.

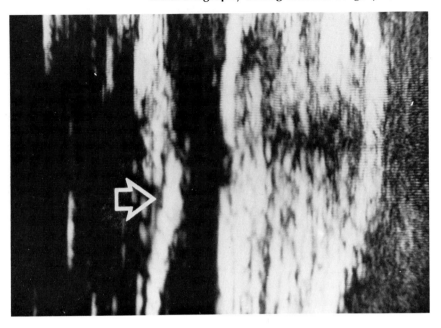

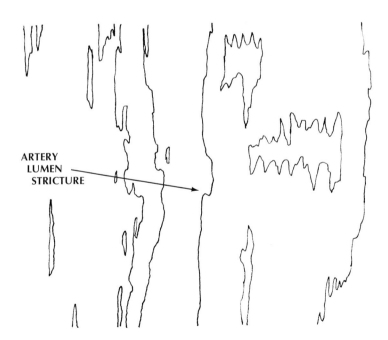

ARTERY
LUMEN
STRICTURE

Fig. 7–9. Sonogram of a longitudinal section of dog aorta shows a stricture (arrow) narrowing the diameter by about 25%.

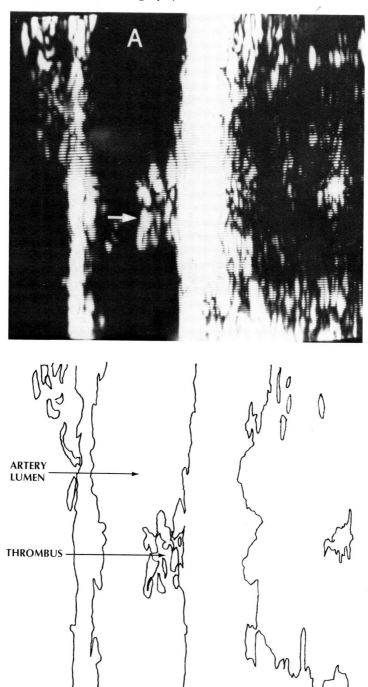

Fig. 7–10. Sonogram of a dog aorta (A) in longitudinal section shows a small thrombus (arrow) attached to the wall.

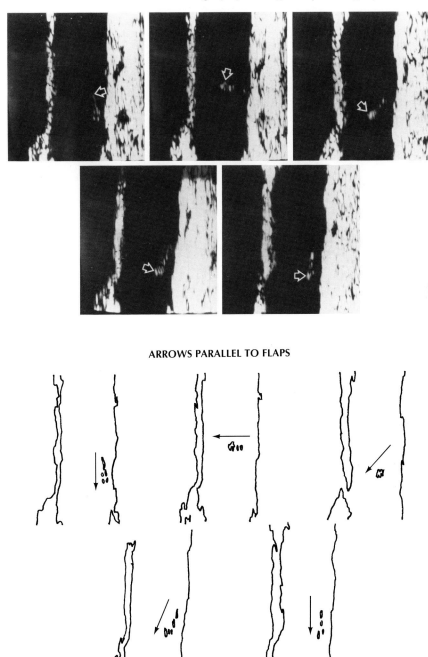

Fig. 7–11. A composite of sonograms showing different positions of the same 5-mm intimal flap in a dog aorta.

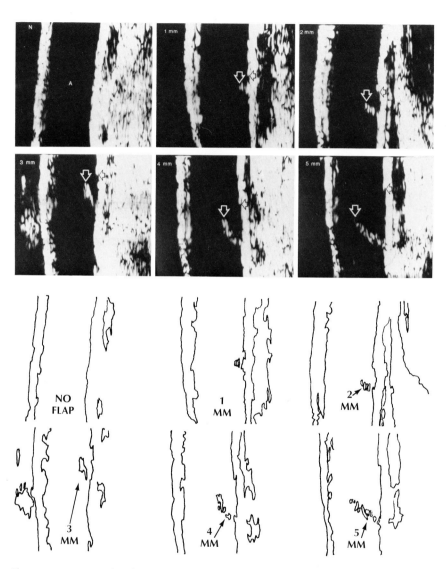

Fig. 7–12. A composite of sonograms of longitudinal sections taken through the dog aorta (A). The upper left view is a normal segment. The remaining sonograms, starting with the middle upper views show different sized flaps (open black arrows) progressing from 1 to 5 millimeters in dimension. The step-off in the intimal defect resulting from dissection of the flaps is shown by the open white arrows.

Figure 7-13 demonstrates a plaque at the carotid bifurcation prior to endarterectomy. Plaques were echogenic and usually produced acoustic shadows of varying density. Figures 7-14 and 7-15 show carotid sites after endarterectomy that appear completely normal. Figures 7-16, 7-17, and 7-18 identify anastomotic sites that are completely open and demonstrate no abnormalities.

Various abnormalities found after reconstruction are shown in Figures 7-19 through 7-23. Figure 7-19 shows a slight stricture at the site of a distal splenorenal venous anastomosis. Because there was no pressure gradient across the anastomosis, the stoma was not revised. This shunt thrombosed in the early postoperative period. Small intimal flaps are seen in Figures 7-20 and 7-21. These occurred at sites of vascular clamp placement and were not considered to be clinically significant and were left undisturbed. The postoperative courses in these patients were uneventful. Figure 7-22 demonstrates an intimal flap, estimated to be 5 to 6 mm in size, in the common carotid artery following an endarterectomy of an innominate-common carotid-internal carotid segment. This flap occurred in a portion of the vessel that underwent blind endarterectomy and was considered too large and too critically located to leave undisturbed. The artery was reopened, and the flap was confirmed and removed. This patient underwent an uneventful recovery.

The intimal flaps observed clinically moved with the pulsatile flow streams in the arteries. This motion was similar to the motion of intimal flaps seen in experimental animals. The ability to discern flap movement significantly improved their detectability and was an important feature of real-time imaging.

The status of arterial dilations may be established by operative ultrasonography. Figure 7-23 shows a section through a mycotic aneurysm that reveals a partial thrombosis.

RESULTS

Operative ultrasound has been employed during 70 vascular operations to examine 128 anastomotic and endarterectomy sites. The operations included 69 arterial procedures and 1 distal splenorenal shunt.

During three operations, operative ultrasound identified the location and extent of atheromatous disease more precisely than did preoperative arteriography. In one patient, a femoropopliteal bypass had been performed for occlusion of the superficial femoral artery. The distal runoff was only marginally satisfactory. However, preoperative arteriography indicated that the plaque extended well into the calf arteries and that an improved runoff could not be obtained without bypass to the distal calf region. Operative ultrasonography performed immediately after completion of the distal anastomosis revealed that the popliteal plaque extended for only about a centi-

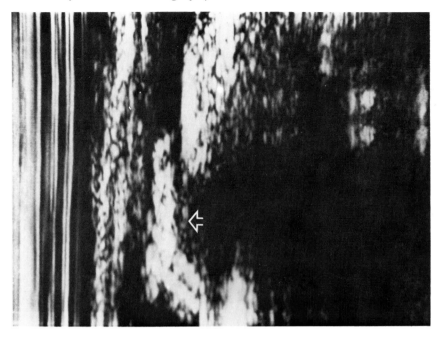

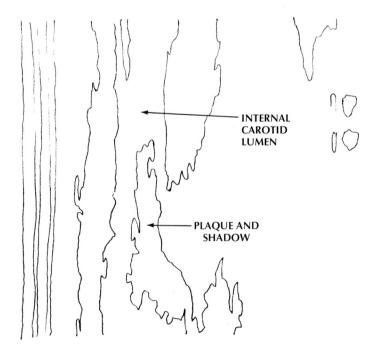

Fig. 7–13. Sonogram of a longitudinal section through an internal carotid artery shows an echogenic plaque (arrow) and acoustic shadow.

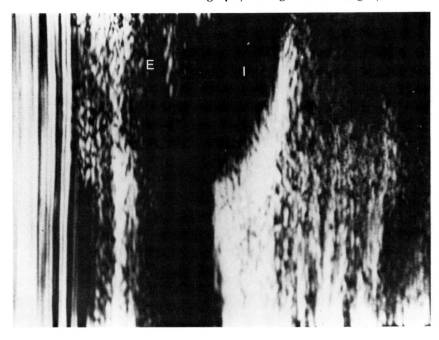

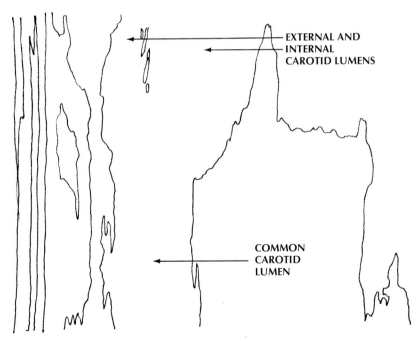

EXTERNAL AND
INTERNAL
CAROTID LUMENS

COMMON
CAROTID
LUMEN

Fig. 7–14.   Sonogram showing a longitudinal section through a carotid bifurcation immediately after endarterectomy. The external (E) and internal (I) carotid arteries are seen without abnormalities.

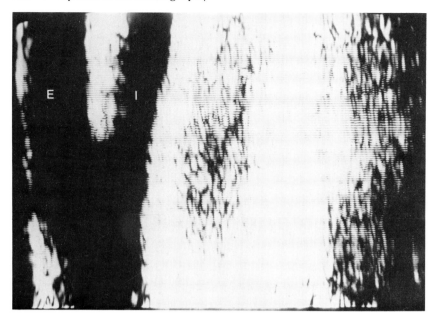

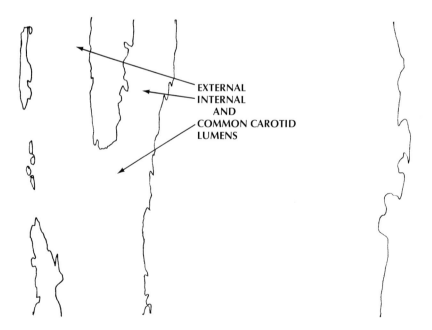

EXTERNAL
INTERNAL
AND
COMMON CAROTID
LUMENS

Fig. 7–15. Sonogram demonstrating a carotid bifurcation after endarterectomy shows the external (E) and internal (I) carotid arteries without intimal or luminal defects.

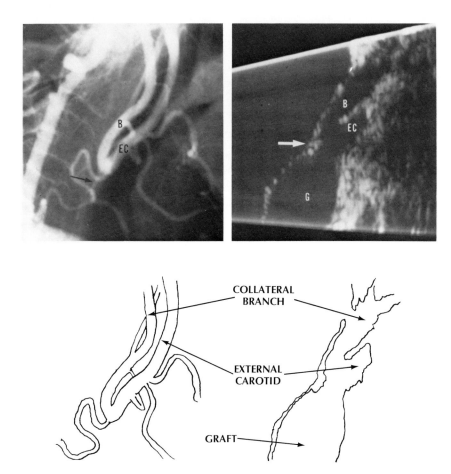

Fig. 7–16. Composite of a preoperative arteriogram (left) showing completely occluded common and internal carotid arteries and the external carotid (EC) filling by means of a collateral branch artery (B). The sonogram (right) shows the same arterial branch (B) and external carotid (EC). A bypass graft (G), seen on the sonogram, connects to the external carotid artery.

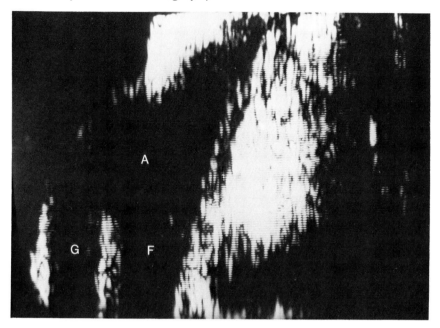

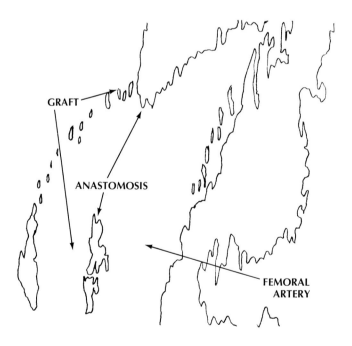

Fig. 7–17. Sonogram showing a through-the-graft section of the proximal anastomosis of a femoropopliteal bypass. The graft (G) joins the femoral artery (F) at a widely open anastomosis (A).

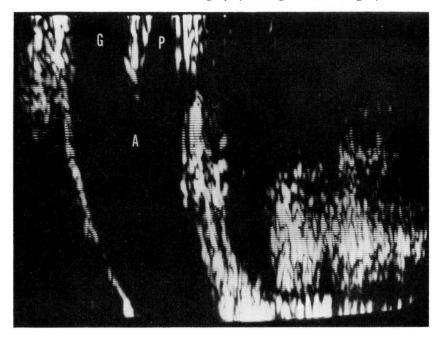

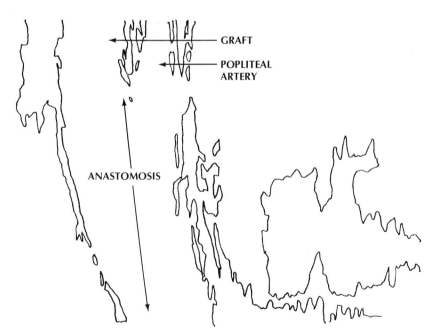

Fig. 7–18. Sonogram showing a through-the-graft section of the distal anastomosis of a femoropopliteal bypass. The graft (G) joins the popliteal artery (P) in an extensive anastomosis (A).

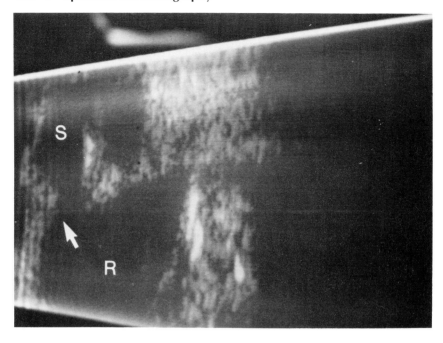

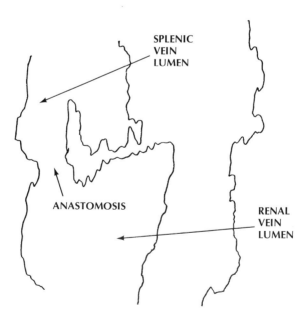

Fig. 7–19. Sonogram showing a section through the anastomosis of a distal splenorenal shunt. The splenic vein (S)-to-renal vein junction (R) demonstrates a slight stricture (arrow).

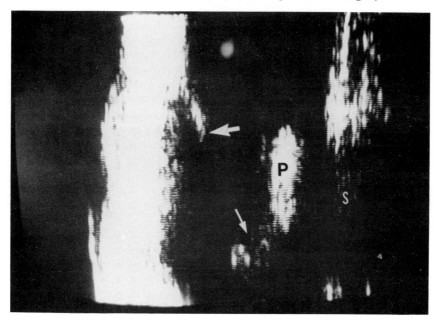

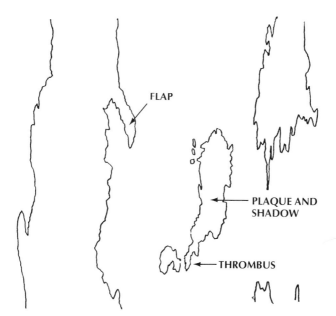

Fig. 7–20. Sonogram of a common femoral artery above a femeropopliteal bypass graft and at the site of application of an occlusive vascular clamp. An atheromatous plaque (P) and acoustic shadows (S) are seen. A thrombus is attached to the lower end of the plaque (lower, small arrow). An intimal flap, approximately 2 to 3 mm in size, is indicated by the upper, larger arrow. The location of the intimal flap corresponds to the placement site for the occlusive clamp.

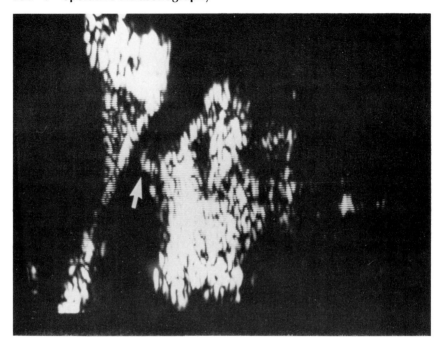

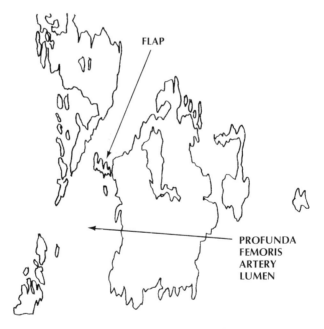

Fig. 7–21. Sonogram showing a longitudinal section through a profunda femoris artery. The arrow points to a 2-mm flap at the site of application of a vascular clamp.

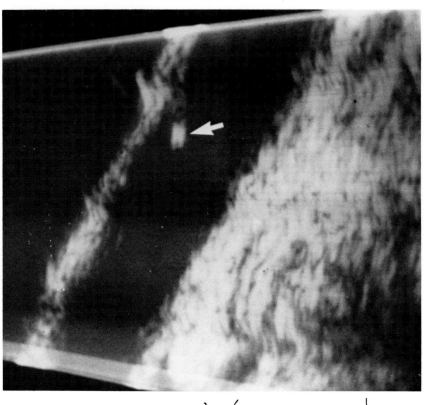

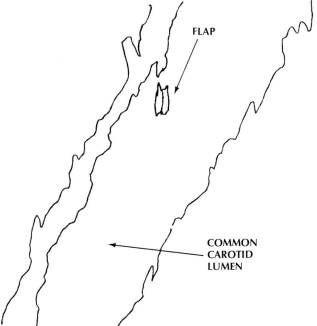

FLAP

COMMON
CAROTID
LUMEN

Fig. 7–22. Sonogram through a common carotid artery after endarterectomy. A 5-mm intimal flap is indicated by the arrow. This vessel was reopened, and the flap was excised.

159

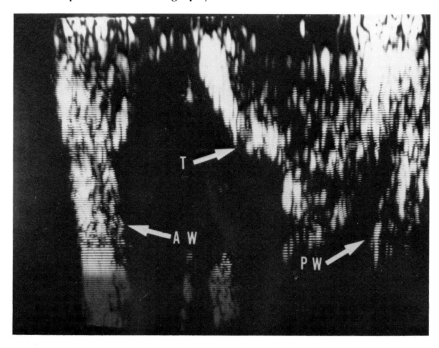

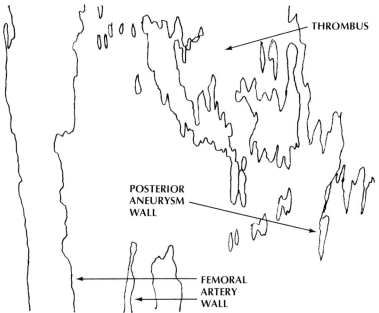

Fig. 7–23. Sonogram showing a section through a mycotic aneurysm in the femoral artery. Arrows point to the anterior wall (AW), posterior wall (PW), and a thrombus (T) within the aneurysm.

meter and that the posterior tibial artery had a good lumen at this point. As a result of this information, a patch-graft angioplasty to widen the lumen was performed immediately distal to the lower anastomosis. This provided a significant improvement in outflow for the bypass graft.

In a second patient with extracranial atherosclerotic disease, preoperative arteriography suggested but did not definitively establish a complete occlusion of an internal carotid artery. Operative ultrasound confirmed complete occlusion. Based on this supportive evidence, an operative decision was made to perform a subclavian external carotid bypass rather than to attempt a carotid endarterectomy.

In a third patient undergoing a popliteal-tibial bypass, two previously unrecognized 5-by-5-mm plaques near the popliteal anastomotic site were identified by operative ultrasound. However, this discovery did not alter management.

In 14 patients, operative ultrasonography revealed a total of 15 vascular defects resulting from reconstructive surgery. There was one small thrombus in a tibial artery following femorotibial bypass. One arterial bypass anastomosis showed a slight stricture. The distal splenorenal shunt also revealed a slight stricture. However, pressure measurements on either side of this anastomosis revealed no pressure gradient. The remaining 12 vascular defects were intimal flaps.

The intimal flaps were observed under one of two circumstances. Either they were associated with an endarterectomy site (carotid or femoral) or they were located at the site of application of occlusive vascular clamps. The flaps ranged in size from 2 to 6 millimeters. All the flaps but one were considered to pose less risk to the patient than arteriotomy for excision. The reasons for these decisions were that the intimal flaps were either too small or not strategically located, meaning that either the vessel was of large caliber compared to the flap or the vessel was functionally not significant.

The single exception, in which an artery was reopened to remove an intimal flap, occurred in a patient who underwent an endarterectomy of the innominate-common carotid-internal carotid segment. This operation was performed through separate arteriotomies in the innominate and in the junction between the right common and internal carotid arteries. The plaque between these incisions was removed by blind dissection. Immediately after arterial closure and restoration of blood flow, operative ultrasound revealed a 5 to 6-mm flap in a portion of the common carotid artery that was not endarterectomized under direct vision. This flap was considered to be clinically significant. For this reason, the artery was reopened, and an 8-by-5-mm intimal flap was excised.

The postoperative course for all 14 patients with discovered postsurgical vascular defects was uneventful except for the patient with the distal splenorenal shunt. In the early postoperative period, this patient developed a thrombosis at the anastomosis site.

CONCLUSIONS

There are two main applications of imaging ultrasound during vascular surgery. The first is to supplement information provided by preoperative arteriography. The second is to detect vascular defects, such as thrombi, strictures, and intimal flaps, immediately after vascular reconstruction and restoration of blood flow but still during the surgical procedure. This is important in assuring the surgeon that potentially harmful defects are not left behind inadvertently. If defects are present, the surgeon should be given an opportunity to make an early decision regarding the appropriateness of vascular re-entry to correct the defects.

Preoperative arteriography is the key to a decision to operate and provides the essential anatomic information on which the operation is based. Occasionally, this information may not be sufficient in two respects. There may be incomplete filling of an arterial segment immediately distal to an obstruction. These situations may be interpreted as obliteration of the lumen or as failure to achieve sufficient retrograde flow of the contrast material to fully demonstrate the postobstructive arterial segment. Furthermore, relating the arteriographic defects with operative findings may be difficult. These occasions were not common. Usually, the combined information provided by preoperative arteriography and the observations at surgery were sufficient to proceed with the operation. However, when this information was insufficient, operative ultrasonography was helpful in assessment and in relating the disorder to anatomic landmarks in the operative field.

The main application of real-time imaging ultrasound during vascular surgery in detecting vascular defects created during the reconstructive procedures. The problem with such defects is the difficulty of early diagnosis during the surgical procedure. Small strictures, thrombi, and intimal flaps may not produce visible or palpable abnormalities immediately after blood flow has been restored. They may, at first, be too inconsequential to cause detectable hemodynamic changes. The first sign of difficulty may be an occlusive complication, which either may cause significant initial damage or may be unrecognized until its effects are fairly advanced. To counter this risk, operative arteriography has been employed to provide early warning of vascular defects.[22-24]

Operative arteriography serves two useful purposes. First, it is capable of detecting vascular defects at the operative site. Second, it provides important information about the distal arterial tree which, because of occlusive disease, may not have been completely visualized with preoperative arteriography. Detailed information about the distal arterial tree is particularly important in lower extremity reconstructions because it may indicate the potential need and feasibility of bypass surgery to the arteries below the knee. This information may also provide an indication of the suitability of the distal arterial tree for more distal bypass surgery at a later date. However, operative arteriography entails risk, especially in carotid surgery. This fact, together with our experimental findings that real-time ultrasound scanning is capable of detecting small defects with a sensitivity that is equivalent to or better than arteriography, prompted us to consider operative ultrasonography as the preferred imaging procedure to detect vascular defects during surgery. This preference would be particularly strong if there were no real need to visualize the distal arterial bed.

During the 70 operations in which ultrasound evaluation was used, vascular defects were found in more than 20% of patients. At the 14 operations in which defects were found, a decision to re-enter to correct the defect was made only once. In the remaining instances, the defects were considered as too slight or were located at sufficiently nonstrategic sites to justify the risk of reclamping and re-entry. These judgments appeared to be valid in all but one patient (who developed an early postoperative complication that was directly attributable to the vascular defect). The fact that so many defects could be correctly regarded as clinically insignificant indicates that operative ultrasound has high sensitivity. This finding corresponds to the high sensitivity encountered in our animal experiments.

A high discovery rate for vascular defects (high sensitivity) has also been described by Lane.[25] This report did not indicate what proportion of positive results was significant enough to warrant re-entry.

Several factors appeared to be associated with the presence of intimal flaps, which were the most common vascular defect found by operative ultrasonography. First, intimal flaps were observed with either endarterectomy or the application of vascular clamps to produce blood flow occlusion. The occurrence of flaps with endarterectomy and not with anastomosis is not surprising. Dissection of an atheromatous plaque can easily produce intimal undermining at the site where the surgeon elects to end the endarterectomy. Normally, great care is exercised to make sure that loose intima is not present and, if present, that it is anchored back to the artery wall.

The occurrence of intimal flaps at sites of clamp occlusion also is not surprising. This finding should re-emphasize the extreme delicacy of atheromatous arteries and the need to use the least traumatic techniques in their manipulation.

A second factor that appeared to be important in our experience was that the only intimal flap that was judged significant enough to warrant re-entry occurred in an arterial segment submitted to endarterectomy without direct vision. This result stresses the usefulness of direct visualization in performing endarterectomy. Furthermore, this occurrence emphasizes the need to be especially thorough with ultrasonic scanning in arterial segments that are endarterectomized under less-than-complete visualization.

Finally, the high sensitivity of operative ultrasonography calls for the establishment of ultrasonic indications for vascular re-entry. These indications must be based on specific findings that indicate significance on the basis of the extent and location of the vascular defects. By the use of such criteria, the vascular surgeon may be rewarded with a greater peace of mind that all is well after vascular closure and with a lower complication rate following vascular reconstruction.

RECOMMENDED APPLICATIONS

1. Operative ultrasonography may be used to supplement information provided by preoperative arteriography. Arterial segments distal to areas of obstruction may be incompletely filled with contrast material. This may preclude an accurate assessment of the extent of the occlusive process. In these instances, operative ultrasound may be employed to survey the exposed portions of the artery and to permit a better examination for atheromatous disease. This examination should be able to relate discovered abnormalities to external anatomic landmarks. Such an ability could be helpful in decisions regarding the site and extent of arteriotomies and types of procedures to perform.

2. Following vascular reconstruction (anastomosis or endarterectomy), operative real-time ultrasound scanning is a useful measure for the detection of vascular defects, such as strictures, thrombi, and intimal flaps. These defects may not be apparent on the basis of inspection or palpation because, initially, they are not hemodynamically significant. However, because they may lead to postoperative thrombosis, one should be aware of their presence.

Experimentally, real-time B-mode ultrasonic scanning compares favorably to arteriography in detecting vascular defects. Clinical evaluation of operative ultrasound also indicates a high sensitivity for the detection of vascular defects. Based on these findings, real-time B-mode ultrasound scanning is recommended as a scanning procedure to search for vascular defects after reconstructive surgery. Such surveillance would be particularly important after endarterectomy, especially if a portion of the procedure was not performed under direct visualization.

CHAPTER 8

NEW AND DEVELOPING USES FOR OPERATIVE ULTRASOUND

Operative ultrasonography has been used in a number of areas in which experience is still insufficient to define its ultimate role. A number of uses are presented in this chapter with a brief description of their rationale, technique, and preliminary results. With time and further development, these uses may become more extensively employed during operation.

FOREIGN BODY EXTRACTION

The localization and removal of foreign bodies is frequently tedious and frustrating because of the difficulty in locating the object. Operative ultrasound has two main advantages in this type of surgery: it may be used in a repeated or prolonged fashion during surgery and imaging sections may be obtained through multiple planes.

The extended use of ultrasonography in varying planes permits localization, depth appraisal, and guidance of an exploring needle to the site of lodgement. The fact that this may be performed in direct reference to visible anatomic landmarks in the operative field greatly facilitates application.

Technique

After the operative site has been prepared and draped, a preliminary ultrasound examination is made through the intact skin. Because of the limitations of penetration of the ultrasound beam, the foreign body cannot be deeper than 3 to 4 centimeters to permit detection. Acoustic coupling is

165

obtained with sterile methylcellulose gel, which is commercially available and is widely used in ophthalmology.

Figure 8-1 shows a preoperative roentgenogram of the hand demonstrating a glass foreign body in the hand. Figure 8-2 depicts the scanning maneuvers used to locate the foreign body. After the foreign body has been located, an exploring needle should be inserted to the site of lodgement. As with the location of renal calculi (see Chap. 6, *Ultrasonography During Renal Surgery*), the exploratory needle may be passed free-hand or with the use of a needle-guide attachment to the transducer-probe. Free-hand passage is best used for relatively large foreign bodies. Use of the needle-guide is recommended for small objects. During passage of the needle employing the guide, the foreign body and the advancing needle are kept under constant surveillance on the monitor screen. Figure 8-3 shows the ultrasonic appearance of the glass foreign body, and Figure 8-4 is a photograph of the specimen after removal.

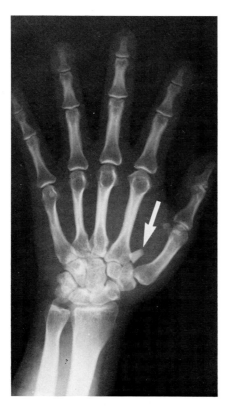 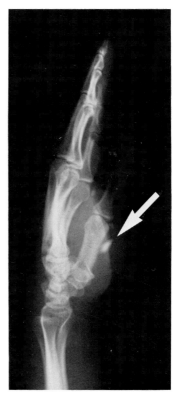

Fig. 8–1. Posteroanterior and lateral roentgenogram of a hand shows an imbedded glass foreign body (arrow).

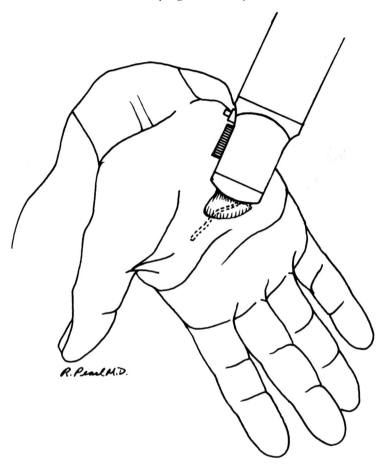

R. Pearl M.D.

Fig. 8–2. Illustration of ultrasound scanning the operative field. Sterile methylcellulose gel was used for acoustic coupling.

Preliminary Results

We have employed ultrasound to locate foreign bodies at operation on five occasions. The technique was helpful in four of these operations. In these instances, ultrasound precisely located the foreign body and assisted in the guidance of a needle to the site of lodgement. The areas of involvement were the calf of the leg, the hand, and the chest wall. The objects were either glass or steel fragments (e.g., portions of a sewing needle).

The failure to localize a foreign body by operative ultrasound occurred with a segment of a sewing needle buried deep in the hand. The steel fragment was lying against the surface of a metacarpal bone. The ultrasonic image of the foreign body was lost in the strong reflective echoes and

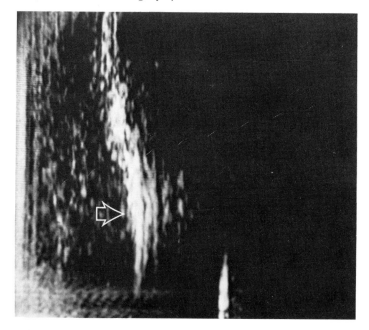

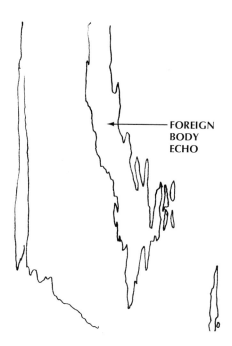

FOREIGN
BODY
ECHO

Fig. 8–3. Sonogram showing an intense echo (arrow) produced by the foreign body.

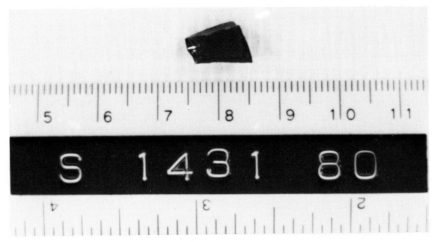

Fig. 8–4. Glass foreign body removed from the hand.

reverberations produced by the bone. This patient may illustrate a fundamental weakness of localizing foreign bodies by ultrasound. Foreign bodies in close proximity to bony structures may be missed. Only those foreign bodies surrounded by soft tissue may be more amenable to ultrasonic localization.

Although each of the foreign bodies in our experience was radiopaque, some foreign bodies (e.g., nonleaded glass or wood) are nonopaque. Operative ultrasound may be especially useful in their extraction.

BRAIN SURGERY

B-mode real-time ultrasonic scanning has been employed during craniotomy for brain tumors. By imaging the tumor after the bone flap has been elevated, the neurosurgeon may obtain precise information about location, size, depth, and consistency (solid or cystic) of the tumor.[26,27]

Technique

Ultrasonography during brain surgery has been performed through intact dura after the bone flap has been elevated. To achieve sufficient depth of sound-beam penetration, the transducer should operate at frequencies below 7.5 MHz. Otherwise, the innermost aspect of the tumors may not be visualized.

Preliminary Results

Real-time B-mode ultrasound scanning during craniotomy has demonstrated both anatomic structure and brain tumors. In brain-tumor imaging, ultrasound has helped to localize lesions and to distinguish solid from cystic tumors.

SOLID ORGAN ABSCESSES

Operative ultrasonography has been used to confirm the presence of abscess in the liver and the spleen. In the liver, the main benefit of ultrasonic scanning has been to localize accurately the abscess and to provide guidance for an exploratory needle. In the spleen, ultrasound has helped to assess the full extent of abscess to determine if a portion of the spleen may be salvaged.

Technique

Ultrasonic scanning for liver abscess and splenic abscess is shown in Figures 8-5 and 8-6. Depending on the depth of the abscess, the position of the transducer-probe may be either at the surface of the organ or withdrawn a few millimeters from the surface.

In the examination of the liver, longitudinal scanning with transverse angulation has been employed along parallel scan paths about a centimeter apart over the suprahepatic and the subhepatic surfaces. When a lesion has been found, transverse scanning has been used to delineate further the extent of the cavity.

The examination of the spleen is performed in a manner similar to ultrasonic scanning of the liver. Less of the splenic surface may be accessible

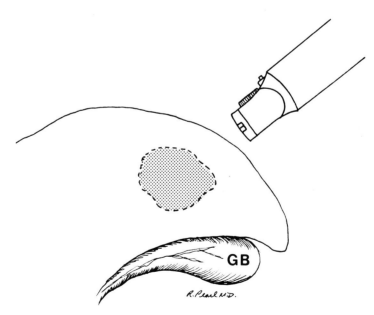

Fig. 8–5.   Illustration of operative liver scanning in search of a liver abscess. GB represents gallbladder.

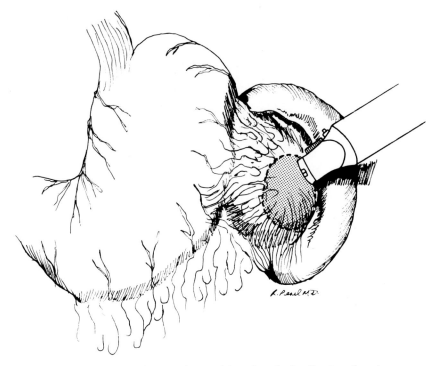

Fig. 8–6. Illustration of an ultrasound scan of the spleen for localization of an abscess.

for transducer-probe placement. For this reason, the operator may have to rely on greater use of longitudinal and transverse angulation to obtain complete visualization of the organ.

Preliminary Results

Operative ultrasound has been employed at four operations for liver abscess. Two of these were amebic and two were pyogenic. Figure 8-7 shows the ultrasonic appearance of both normal liver and abscess. All liver abscesses demonstrated relatively sonolucent cavities with some internal echoes. Ultrasonography localized the abscesses at all operations and helped to provide assurance of the absence of multiple abscesses. All patients did well postoperatively.

Operative ultrasonography has been used at two operations for splenic abscesses. Both were pyogenic and one was secondary to splenic emboliza-tion in a patient with subacute bacterial endocarditis. One patient had a single, large, centrally placed abscess cavity, whereas the patient with endocarditis showed multiple abscesses (Fig. 8-8). The abscess cavities all appeared relatively sonolucent compared to adjacent splenic tissue. In both patients, the size and extent of the abscesses precluded any possibility of

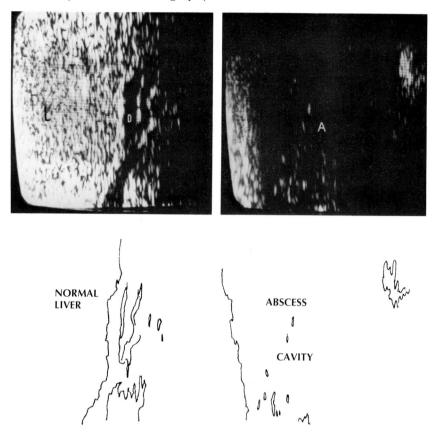

Fig. 8–7. Composite of two sonograms obtained from the same liver. The view on the left shows normal liver (L) tissue and a liver duct (D). The view on the right shows a thin rim of liver tissue and an abscess cavity (A) with only a few internal echoes.

salvaging a portion of the organs. Splenectomies were performed, and the postoperative course of both patients was uneventful.

Operative ultrasound may be useful in permitting partial splenectomy with salvage of a splenic remnant. This could occur if an abscess was found to be localized near one pole and the remainder of the organ was shown to be normal.

ENDOCRINE SURGERY

Operative ultrasonography has been used in parathyroid,[28] adrenal, and pancreatic surgery for Zollinger-Ellison tumor.[29] The purpose of this utilization has been to determine the ultrasonic features of endocrine tumors and to evaluate the possible role of operative ultrasonography in helping to find tumors that are small and difficult to localize.

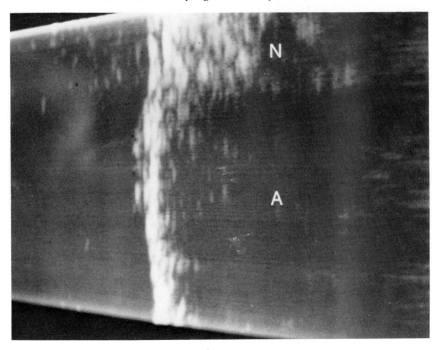

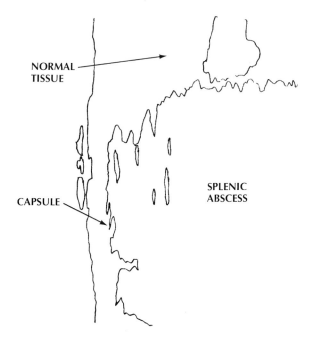

Fig. 8–8. Sonogram showing a longitudinal section through a spleen. Normal splenic tissue is at N. An abscess cavity is seen at A.

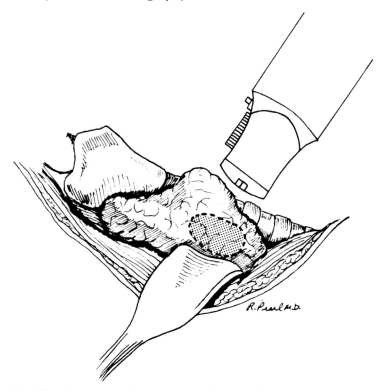

Fig. 8–9. Illustration of operative ultrasonography in search of a parathyroid adenoma.

Technique

The search for parathyroid tumors has been conducted after the strap muscles of the neck have been retracted to expose the thyroid gland (Fig. 8-9). Ultrasonic scanning has been performed through the thyroid gland and into surrounding tissue using longitudinal scanning with transverse angulation. Parallel scan paths should be ½ to 1 centimeter apart.

Examination of the adrenal regions involves scanning over the posterior peritoneum over a wide surface to characterize any obvious tumors and to search for multiple lesions (Fig. 8-10). Examination of the pancreas for an endocrine tumor is conducted in a manner described previously (see Chap. 5, *Ultrasonography During Pancreatic Surgery*). The distance between parallel scan paths should be as short as possible to make certain that small tumors within the pancreas are not missed.

Preliminary Results

Ultrasonography has been used at four operations for primary hyperparathyroidism. In three of these, ultrasound helped to locate adenomas ranging from 1 to 2 centimeters in size (Figs. 8-11 and 8-12). In a fourth patient,

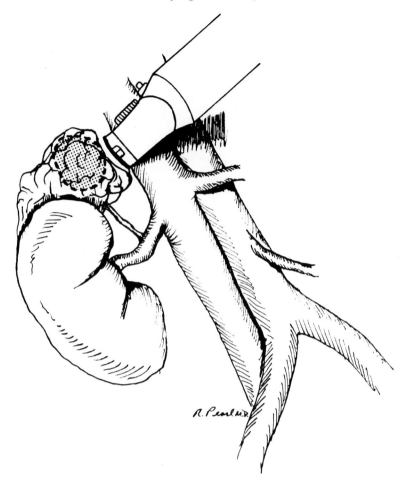

Fig. 8–10.   Illustration of ultrasound scanning of an adrenal tumor.

ultrasonography, which was conducted only over the region of the thyroid gland, did not locate an adenoma that was ultimately found in a retropharangeal position. All parathyroid adenomas were relatively sonolucent when compared to the adjacent thyroid tissue. Although none of the ultrasonically discovered adenomas was particularly small or atypically placed, operative ultrasound apparently did facilitate and shorten the search process.

Ultrasonography has been performed at one operation for a right adrenal tumor. This tumor was large and readily apparent on preoperative arteriography and during the operation. During ultrasonography, the tumor proved to be relatively sonolucent (Fig. 8-13). The right adrenal gland was removed, and the pathologic diagnosis was adrenal adenoma.

A patient with Zollinger-Ellison syndrome diagnosed by history of previous peptic ulceration and markedly elevated serum gastrin levels revealed

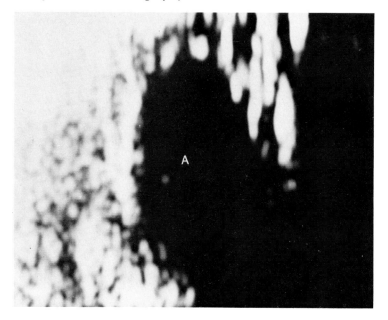

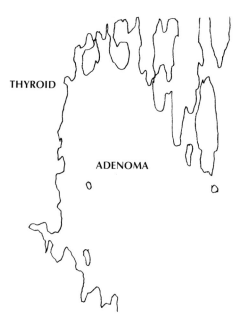

Fig. 8–11. Sonogram showing a sonolucent parathyroid adenoma (A) posterior to and partially embedded in the thyroid gland, which is more echogenic than the adenoma.

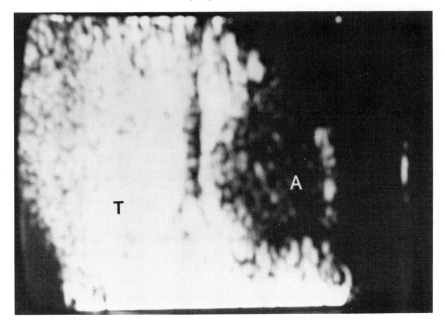

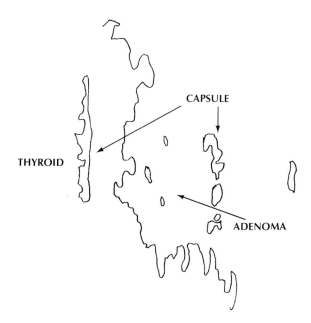

Fig. 8–12. Sonogram showing a parathyroid adenoma (A) deep to the thyroid gland (T). The adenoma is relatively sonolucent. The capsule of the adenoma shows increased echogenicity.

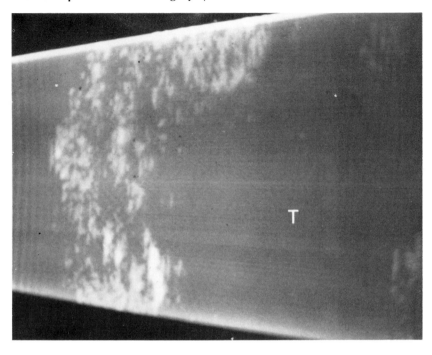

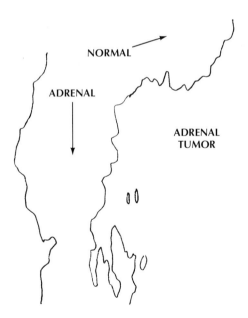

Fig. 8–13.   Sonogram of an adrenal adenoma. The normal adrenal tissue is echogenic (at left), whereas the adenoma (T) is sonolucent.

a small tumor on the surface of the pancreas at the junction of the body and tail. This tumor was ultrasonically scanned at operation and found to be sonolucent. A partial pancreatectomy was performed. Pathologic diagnosis was islet cell tumor (benign) associated with diffuse microadenomatosis.

It is noteworthy that all endocrine tumors ultrasonically scanned during operation were sonolucent when compared to surrounding tissue. This sonolucency has been observed in ultrasonography of parathyroid adenomas.[28] If sonolucency proves to be a consistent finding, operative ultrasonography may be useful in detecting less obvious tumors than those encountered in our experience to date. Sonolucency may be distinctive enough to discover smaller lesions in unusual locations and within the substance of other organs, such as parathyroid adenomas within the thyroid gland and small islet cell tumors within the pancreas. More experience is needed to assess this possibility further.

REFERENCES

1. Sigel, B, et al.: Intraoperative ultrasonic visualization of biliary calculi. Curr Surg, 36:158, 1979.
2. White, DN: Ultrasound in Medical Diagnosis. Kingston, Ontario, Ultramedison, 1976.
3. Wells, PNT: Biomedical Ultrasonics. London, Academic Press, 1977.
4. Bronson, NR: Development of a simple B-scan ultrasonoscope. Trans Am Ophthalmol Soc, 70:365, 1972.
5. Berci, G, and Hamlin, JA: Operative Biliary Radiology. Baltimore, Williams & Wilkins, 1981.
6. Holmin, T, et al.: Selective or routine intraoperative cholangiography: a cost-effectiveness analysis. World J Surg, 4:315, 1980.
7. Skillings, JC, Williams, JS, and Hinshaw, JR: Cost-effectiveness of operative cholangiography. Am J Surg, 137:26, 1979.
8. Sigel, B, et al.: Real-time ultrasonography during biliary surgery. Radiology, 137:531, 1980.
9. Lane RJ, and Glazer, G: Intraoperative B-mode ultrasound scanning of the extra-hepatic biliary system and pancreas. Lancet II, 8190:334, 1980.
10. Sigel, B, et al.: Ultrasonic imaging during biliary and pancreatic surgery. Am J Surg, 141:84, 1981.
11. Cattell, RB, and Warren, KW: Surgery of the pancreas. Philadelphia, Saunders, 1954.
12. Schlegel, JU, Diggdon, P, and Cuellar, J: The use of ultrasound for localizing renal calculi. J Urol, 86:367, 1961.
13. Cook, JH, and Lytton, B: Intraoperative localization of renal calculi during nephrolithotomy by ultrasound scanning. J Urol, 117:543, 1977.
14. Lytton, B, and Cook, JH: Intraoperative ultrasound. In: Ultrasound in Urology. Edited by MI Resnick, and RC Saunders. Baltimore, Williams & Wilkins, 1979.
15. Sigel, B, et al.: Ultrasonic scanning during operation for renal calculi. J Urol. In press.
16. Sigel, B, et al.: Ultrasonic imaging during vascular surgery. Arch Surg. In press.
17. Mercier, LA, et al.: High-resolution ultrasound arteriography: a comparison with carotid angiography. In Non-invasive Diagnostic Techniques in Vascular Surgery. Edited by EF Bernstein. St. Louis, C.V. Mosby, 1978.
18. Coelho, JCU, et al.: Detection of arterial defects by real-time ultrasound scanning during vascular surgery: an experimental study. J Surg Res, 30:535, 1981.
19. Coelho, JCU, et al.: An experimental evaluation of arteriography and imaging ultrasonography in detecting arterial defects at operation. J Surg Res. In press.
20. Sigel, B, et al.: Ultrasonography of blood during stasis and coagulation. Invest Radiol, 16:71, 1981.
21. Sigel, B, et al.: Effect of plasma proteins and temperature on echogenicity of blood. Invest Radiol. In press.
22. Dardik, II, et al.: Routine intraoperative angiography. Arch Surg, 110:184, 1975.
23. Plecha, FR, and Pories, WJ: Intraoperative angiography in the immediate assessment of arterial reconstruction. Arch Surg, 105:902, 1972.
24. Rosental, JJ, Gaspar, MR, and Movius, HJ: Intraoperative arteriography in carotid thromboendarterectomy. Arch Surg, 106:806, 1973.
25. Lane, RJ: Intraoperative B-mode scanning. J Clin Ultrasound, 8:427, 1980.
26. Rubin, JM, et al.: Intraoperative ultrasound examination of the brain. Radiology, 137:831, 1980.
27. Voorhies, RM, and Patterson, RH: Preliminary experience with intraoperative ultrasonographic localization of brain tumors. Radiology/Nuclear Medicine Magazine, October, 1980.
28. Sigel, B, et al.: Identification of a parathyroid adenoma by operative ultrasonography. Arch Surg, 116:234, 1981.
29. Sigel, B, et al.: Detection of pancreatic tumors by ultrasound during surgery. Arch Surg (In press).
30. Knight, PR, et al.: Operative use of ultrasonics in cholelithiasis. Lancet i:1023, 1963.
31. Eiseman, B, et al.: Localization of common duct stones by ultrasound. Arch Surg 91:195, 1965.
32. Hayaski, S., et al.: Ultrasonic diagnosis of breast tumor and cholelithiasis. West J Surg, 70:34, 1962.

INDEX

Page numbers in *italics* indicate figures; numbers followed by "t" indicate tables.

Acoustic impedance, 10–11, 129
Acoustic lens(es), 19–20, *20*, 26
Acoustic shadow, 36
Acoustic window, 46, *47*
Adrenal. See *Ultrasound, operative, endocrine*
Air bubbles, 31
American Institute of Ultrasound in Medicine, 30
A-mode, 12, *12*
Angulation, longitudinal, of transducer-probe. See *Scanning maneuver(s)*
transverse, of transducer-probe. See *Scanning maneuver(s)*
Arcing, 138, *139*. See also *Scanning maneuver(s)*
Arterial surgery. See *Ultrasound, operative, vascular*
Arteriography, operative, 162–163
Arteriosclerosis. See *Ultrasound, operative, vascular*
Axial resolution, 22, *22*

Backscattering, 5, 9. See also *Scattering* and *Sound reflection*
Bile duct calculi. See *Ultrasound, operative, of biliary tract, bile duct evaluation of*
Biliary surgery. See *Ultrasound, operative, of biliary tract*
Biopsy, ultrasound guided, 89–90, *91*
B-mode, 13–16, *14*
bistable, 14
compound, 14–15, *15*
real-time, 15–16
B-mode real-time system. See *Pulse processing system*

Cathode-ray tube, 14
Cavitation, 30
Cholangiography, operative, 65–66, 79t, 82–83
Coaxial cable, 16, *17*, 42
Common bile duct localization. See *Ultrasound, operative, of biliary tract, anatomic orientation*
Control, sensitivity, 27, 33, 42
Converter, video scan, 29
Coupling, acoustic, 32, 44–45, *44*. See also *Sound medium*

db. See *decibel*
Decibel, 10
Defect(s), vascular. See *Ultrasound, operative, vascular*
Density, defined, 2
Doppler effect principle, 8
Doppler ultrasound velocity detection, 8
Dynamic range, 27–28

Echoe(s), 14
Echogenicity, 12
Efficiency, 79t, 81
Elasticity, defined, 2
Electric current leakage, 31
Experiment(s), acoustic shadow, 35–36, *35*
angulation, 33–35, *34*
echogenicity, 35–36, *35*
focal distance, 37, *38*
ranging, 33–35, *34*
resolution, lateral, 37, *37*. See also *Resolution, lateral*
superior-inferior orientation, 36–37, *36*

183

Flap(s), intimal. See *Ultrasound, operative, vascular*
Fluid, coupling, 37–38. See also *Coupling, acoustic*
Focal distance, 37
Focused transducer(s), 19
Foreign body(ies). See *Ultrasound, operative, foreign body extraction*
Frequency, resonant, 7
Frequency shift, 8

Gallbladder, calculi detection in. See *Ultrasound, operative, of biliary tract, gallbladder content assessment and*
Geometry of transmission and reflective images, definitions and differences, 17–18, *18*
Gray-scale, 27–28
Gray-scale B-mode imaging, defined, 14

Heat, 30
Hertz, 2. See also *Sound, frequency of*
Huygen's principle, defined, 7

Image(s). See specific types of images
Imaging reflective ultrasound, principles of, 9–12
Imaging reflective ultrasound system(s), 12–16
Instrumentation, 25–38, *30*
deployment of, at operation, 42–43, *43*
Interference. See *Sound wave(s), interference of*

Liver. See *Ultrasound, operative, of solid organ abscesses*

Methylcellulose, 32. See also *Coupling, acoustic*
M-mode, 10
diagrams of, 12–13, *13*
Monitor(s), orientation of, 45–46, *45, 46, 47*
oscilloscope, cathode-ray, 27
television, 27, 29
types of, 27
video, 28. See also *Monitors, television*

Needle guidance, ultrasonic, 89–90, *91,* 100, 124, 125, *125*

One-dimensional system(s), 12–13. See also *A-mode; M-mode*
Oscilloscope, cathode-ray, 29. See also *Cathode-ray tube; Monitor(s)*

Pancreas, abscess of. See *Ultrasound, operative, of pancreas, inflammatory disease*

islet-cell tumors of. See *Ultrasound, operative, endocrine*
Pancreatic tumor(s). See *Ultrasound, operative, of pancreas*
Pancreatitis. See *Ultrasound, operative, of pancreas*
Parathyroid. See *Ultrasound, operative, endocrine*
Penetration, factors related to, 23
Periampullary tumor(s). See *Ultrasound, operative, of pancreatic tumors*
Piezoelectric effect, 7–8, *8*
Piezoelectric transducer(s), 7–8, *8,* 9, *9*
Predictive value, of negative or positive test, 79t, 81
Prevalence, 79t, 81
Probe, 16, *17*
Pseudocyst(s), of pancreas. See *Ultrasound, operative, of pancreas, inflammatory disease*
Pulse processing system, 26–29
Bronson and Turner, 27–28, *28*
PS-100-B, 28–29, *29*

Range, defined, 17, *18*
Range resolution. See *Axial resolution*
Range setting, 33, 42
Rate of echo distance changes, 10. See also *M-mode*
Real-time, B-mode, types of transducers, 15–16
Reception rate, 9
Reflection and acoustic impedance, 10–11
Reflective image(s), 17
geometry of, 17–18, *18*
Refraction, 6
Renal calculi. See *Ultrasound, operative, renal*
Renal surgery. See *Ultrasound, operative, renal*
Repetition rate, 23, 33
Reproduction, photography, 27
video tape, 27
Resolution, axial, defined, 20, *20*
factors determining, 23
lateral, 21–22, *21*
defined, 20, *20*
Rouleaux formation, 141

Safety, 29–31
Scanners, "small parts," defined, 26
Scanning. See also *Ultrasound, operative*
defined, 14
longitudinal, of transducer-probe. See *Scanning maneuver(s)*
transverse, of transducer-probe. See *Scanning maneuver(s)*
whole body, 23

Scanning maneuver(s), 46-52, *49–52*
  images produced by, 48–52, *49–52*
  types of, 48, *49*, 138, *139*
Scanning motion, 16
Scattering, 4–5, *5*, 9. See also *Sound reflection*
Sensitivity, 80–81, *79t*
Sonolucency, 14
Sound, defined, 1–3
  directionality of, 18
    frequency and, 3–4, *3*
  frequency of, 1, 2
  intensity of, 27–28, 32. See also *Decibel and Sound amplitude*
  interaction of, in a medium, 3–7
  properties of, 1–3
  transmission of, in a medium, 3–7
  velocity of. See *Sound velocity*
  wavelength of, 1, 2
Sound absorption, 11, 29
  causative factors, 11
  milliwatts, 30
Sound amplification, 33
Sound amplitude, 9
  measurement of, 10
Sound attenuation, defined, 11
Sound beam, far field of, 18–19, *19*
  focal length of, 20, *20*
  focal range of, 20, *20*
  near field of, 18–19, *19*
Sound beam focusing, 19, *20*
Sound beam width, 18–20, *19*
Sound echo, 9
Sound energy intensity. See *Sound amplitude*
Sound medium, 2, 31
  propagation velocity and, 2
Sound properties, 3
Sound pulse, 9, 22
Sound reflection, 9, 10
  defined, 3
  equation for, 10
Sound velocity, 10
  in air, 2
  in bone, 2
  in soft tissue, 2
  in water, 2
Sound wave(s), cancellation of, 6, 7
  interference of, 6–7, *6*
  phase relation of, 7
  reinforcement of, 6, 7
Specificity, *79t*, 80–81
Specular reflection, 4–5, *4*, 9. See also *Sound reflection*
Spleen. See *Ultrasound, operative, of solid organ abscesses*
Sterilization, technique and temperature limits of. See *Transducer-probe sterility*
Storage oscilloscope, 14

Stricture(s), vascular. See *Ultrasound, operative, vascular*

Technique(s). See *Ultrasound, operative*
  general, 39–52
Thrombi. See *Ultrasound, operative, vascular*
Time and distance relation, 10
Time-gain compensation, 11–12, *12*, 32
Tissue motion, 16
Tissue penetration, 33
Transducer(s), 18, 25–26, 31
  linear array, 15, *16*
  mechanical sector scanning, 15, *16*, 25
  phased array, 15, *16*
  piezoelectric, 7–8, *8*, 9, *9*
Transducer function, 18–20
Transducer-probe(s), 16, *17*, 31, *32*. See also *Transducer(s)*
  disposable sterile cover of, 41–42, *41*
  scanning with. See *Scanning maneuver(s)*
Transducer-probe placement, 43–46, *44–47*
  "dry," 43–44, 54, 122, *123*, 137, *139–141*
  "wet," 45–46
Transducer-probe sterility, 39–41, *40*
Transmission image(s), geometry of, 17–18, *18*
Two-dimensional system(s), 13–16. See also *B-mode*

Ultrasonography, operative, 23
Ultrasound, basics of, 1–23
  defined, 2
  types of, diagnostic, 8–9
  Doppler, 8
  high-frequency, 23
  imaging reflective, 9, *9*
  operative, brain, 169
    defined, vii
    during nephrolithotomy, 122–131
      error avoidance in, 129–131, *132*
      findings in, 126–131, *127–129*, *132*
      needle guidance in, 124–125, *125*
      technique of, 122–126, *123*, *125*
    endocrine, 172–179
      preliminary results of, 174–179, *176–178*
      technique for, 174, *174*, *175*
    foreign body extraction, 165–169
      preliminary results of, 167–169, *166*, *168*, *169*
      technique for, 165–166, *167*
    new and developing uses, 165–179
    of biliary tract, 53–83
      anatomic orientation for, 53–55, *54*, *56*
      bile duct evaluation of, 65–82, *66–71*, *73–77*, *79t*
      technique for, 66–68, *66–69*

Ultrasound, basics of, operative, brain (Cont.)
  bile duct findings in, 69–77, *70, 71,
    73–77*
  conclusions from, 82
  gallbladder content assessment and,
    55–65, *57, 59–64*
  indications for, 53
  recommended applications for, 82–83
  results of, 78–82, 79t
  of pancreas, 85–119
    conclusions from, 117–118
    indications for, 85
    inflammatory disease and, findings of,
      100–105, *102–104, 106–113*
    technique for, 98–100, *98–101*
    normal, findings of, 86–89, *87, 88*
      technique for, 86, *86*
    recommended applications of,
      118–119
    results of, 105–117
    tumor distinction from inflammation,
      89
  of pancreatic tumors, findings of, 90–97,
    92–96
    technique for, 89–90, *90, 91*
    uses of, 89
  of solid organ abscesses, 170–172
    preliminary results of, 171–172, *172,
      173*
    technique for, 170–171, *170,* 171
  renal, 121–134
    conclusions from, 133
    indications for, 121
    normal findings from, 126, *127*
    recommended application of, 134
    results of, 131–133
  vascular, 135–164
    conclusions from, 162–164
    during surgery, 136–149
    experimental background for, 136,
      141–142, *144–148*
    findings in, 141–149, *143–148,
      150–160*
    indications for, 135, 137
    normal, findings in, 141, *143*
    recommended applications for, 164
    results of, 149–161
    technique for, 137–141, *138–142*
  transmitted, 11
Ultrasound equipment. See *Instrumentation*
Ultrasound image(s), characteristics of,
    16–23
  interpretation of, 33–38
  orientation of, 33–38
Urologic surgery. See *Ultrasound, operative,
    renal*

Vascular surgery. See *Ultrasound, operative,
    vascular*

Wave(s), longitudinal, 1, *2*
Window, probe, 34

X-ray image(s), 17

Zero crossing(s), 22
Zollinger-Ellison tumor. See *Ultrasound,
    operative, endocrine*